McGraw-Hill Education

5 NLN PAX-RN

PRACTICE TESTS

McGraw-Hill Education

5 NLN PAX-RN

PRACTICE TESTS

Joseph Brennan

New York   Chicago   San Francisco   Athens   London   Madrid
Mexico City   Milan   New Delhi   Singapore   Sydney   Toronto

1 2 3 4 5 6 7 8 9 10   LHS   25 24 23 22 21 20

ISBN   978-1-260-46237-1
MHID   1-260-46237-4

e-ISBN   978-1-260-46238-8
e-MHID   1-260-46238-2

The NLN PAX-RN is produced by the National League for Nursing, which was not involved in the production of, and does not endorse, this product.

McGraw-Hill products are available at special quantity discounts to use as premiums and sales promotions or for use in corporate training programs. To contact a representative, please visit the Contact Us pages at www.mhprofessional.com.

Contents

Introduction

FORMAT OF THE TEST

The NLN PAX-RN is administered by the National League for Nursing, a leading professional organization for nurse faculty and others involved in nursing education. It is designed to measure your abilities in the academic areas that are central to nursing education. The NLN exam is a traditional paper-and-pencil test. All of the questions on the NLN PAX-RN exam are multiple-choice items, each with four answer choices. The format of the test is shown below.

Section	Number of Questions	Time Allowed	Content
Verbal Ability	60	40 minutes	Word knowledge, reading comprehension
Mathematics	40	40 minutes	Arithmetic, basic algebra, geometry, graphs, and data interpretation
Science	60	40 minutes	High-school level biology, chemistry, physics, and earth science
Total	**160**	**2 hours**	

HOW THE TEST IS SCORED

For each section of the NLN PAX-RN exam, you receive a raw score based on how many items you answered correctly. Some questions on the exam are included for experimental reasons and are therefore not scored. As a result, the highest possible scores for each section are as follows: Verbal Ability, 60; Mathematics, 40; and Science, 60. You will also receive a composite score that is a weighted combination of your scores on the separate test sections. Composite scores may range from 0 to 200. In addition, you receive percentile scores for each test section and for the test as a whole. These scores are developed using a statistical process. They show what portion of a so-called norms group of similar test-takers earned raw scores that are lower than yours. For example, if you earned a raw score of 52 on the Verbal Ability section with a corresponding percentile score of 85, that means that 85 percent of the test-takers in the norms group earned raw scores that were lower than yours. The NLN says that for each section, percentiles ranging from about 40 to 60 indicate average performance on the exam.

Note that there is no official passing score on this exam. The schools that require applicants to take the NLN PAX-RN establish their own criteria about what scores are considered acceptable for admission.

TYPES OF QUESTIONS
Verbal Ability

On the NLN PAX-RN exam, the Verbal Ability questions are of two types.

First, there are vocabulary questions that test your understanding of specific words. These questions may look like this:

1. The candidates engaged in an *acrimonious* debate.
   Acrimonious means
   a. polite.
   b. public.
   c. meaningless.
   d. combative.

Answer: d. *Acrimonious* means "combative."

The second type of Verbal Ability question is reading comprehension. In this type of question, you are given a reading passage of 400 to 500 words. The passage is usually on a topic in science or medicine. Following the passage are six questions about its content. Each question has four answer choices. You must pick the best answer choice based on your understanding of the passage. Here is an example:

The "food pyramid" is a visual representation of how the different food groups can be combined to form a healthy diet. Although it has been a vital part of dietary guidelines for years, the pyramid is constantly undergoing analysis and revision as additional studying is done in nutritional fields. Recently, the pyramid has undergone another change regarding the unique dietary needs of seniors.

According to an article published in the January 2008 issue of the *Journal of Nutrition*, modifications in the pyramid for older adults include an emphasis on fiber and calcium, as well as on vitamins D and B12. By incorporating these changes, the pyramid now indicates that the nutrients found in a person's routine daily consumption typically are not enough for seniors. Seniors need supplementation.

As people age, they tend to move less and thus need fewer calories to maintain their weight. Because seniors tend to eat a more limited amount, dietitians urge them to choose wisely. They are urged to eat nutrient-rich meals featuring such food as fruits, vegetables, low-fat dairy products, and high-fiber whole grains.

Some experts recommend that older people purchase packaged versions of perishables because such foods last longer than the fresh kind. For example, dried and frozen fruit have a much longer shelf life, as do frozen or canned vegetables. Having a supply of these in the cupboard means fewer trips to the grocery store and less risk of running out of nutritional snacks.

The newly designed pyramid also focuses on the importance for older people of ingesting adequate amounts of fluids on a daily basis. This helps ensure proper digestion and prevent any possibility of dehydration.

Finally, the revised pyramid includes information on incorporating exercise and other physical activities into the lives of older adults. Suggestions include swimming, walking, or simple yard work. Because recent reports have stated that obesity levels for people older than 70 years of age are climbing, performing some type of regular exercise is more essential than ever.

1. The best title for this selection is
   a. America's Seniors Need Exercise.
   b. A New Food Pyramid for Seniors.
   c. Finding Supplementation for Aging.
   d. Dietary Changes in Older Americans.

2. The purpose of updating the food pyramid as described in the passage is to
   a. change how seniors eat.
   b. increase food supplement sales.
   c. encourage people to eat more fruit.
   d. convince older people to start swimming.

3. The passage says that seniors should support their digestion by
   a. taking vitamin D.
   b. eating fewer calories.
   c. drinking adequate fluids.
   d. incorporating some exercise into their regular routine.

4. Dried and frozen fruit is often recommended by dietitians because it is
   a. delicious.
   b. easier to store.
   c. more nutritional than fresh fruit.
   d. known to have a much longer shelf life.

5. The reason that the author of the passage suggests exercise such as swimming, walking, and yard work is because those activities are
   a. ways to interact with other people.
   b. things that can be done alone.
   c. low impact in nature and relatively safe.
   d. useless for burning up calories.

6. The author's purpose in writing this passage was primarily to
   a. alert people to the different dietary needs of seniors.
   b. encourage students to study the pyramid's requirements.
   c. inform nurses about what supplements are most essential.
   d. educate physicians on the differences between dried and fresh fruit.

Answers: 1. b 2. a 3. c 4. d 5. c 6. a

Mathematics

The questions in the Mathematics section of the test are also multiple-choice items with four answer choices. Here is an example:

1. The number 1,200 is what percent of 1,500?
   a. 20 percent
   b. 40 percent
   c. 60 percent
   d. 80 percent

Answer: d. The number 1,200 is 80 percent, or 80%, of 1,500.

Science

The questions in the Science portion of the exam are likewise multiple-choice items. Here is an example:

1. Which of the following transports oxygen in human blood?
   a. Phagocytes and white blood cells
   b. Hemoglobin in red blood cells
   c. Platelets
   d. Lymph from lymph nodes

Answer: b. Hemoglobin in the red blood cells transports oxygen in human blood.

Note that some of the questions in the Science portion of the exam include tables, charts, or illustrations. Sometimes two or more questions are based on the same chart or illustration.

Test-Taking Tips

This chapter presents some general test-taking strategies that can help you gain valuable points when you take your test. At the end of the chapter, you will also find some useful tips that can help you on test day.

GENERAL TEST-TAKING STRATEGIES

Take Advantage of the Multiple-Choice Format

All of the questions on the nursing school entrance exams are in multiple-choice format, which you have undoubtedly seen many times before. That means that for every question, the correct answer is right in front of you. All you have to do is pick it out from among three incorrect choices called *distracters*. Consequently, you can use the process of elimination to rule out incorrect answer choices. The more answers you rule out, the easier it is to make the right choice.

Answer Every Question

On these exams, there is no penalty for choosing a wrong answer. Therefore, if you do not know the answer to a question, you have nothing to lose by guessing. So make sure that you answer every question. If you are taking one of the paper-and-pencil exams and find that you are running out of time, make sure to enter an answer for the questions that you have not tackled. With luck, you may be able to pick up a few extra points, even if your guesses are totally random.

Answer All of the Easy Problems First, Then Tackle the Hard Ones

Keep in mind that these tests all have specific time limits. There is not much time to spend trying to figure out the answers to harder problems, so skip them and come back to them later. There are three reasons why you should do this:

➤ Every question counts the same in the scoring of the exam. That means that you are better off spending time answering the easier questions, where you are sure to pick up points.

➤ Later on in the test you might come to a question or a set of answer choices that jogs your memory and helps you to go back and answer the question you skipped.

➤ By answering the easier questions, you will build your confidence and get into a helpful test-taking rhythm. Then when you go back to a question you skipped, you may find that it is not as hard as you first thought.

Make Educated Guesses

What differentiates great test takers from merely good ones is the ability to guess in a way that maximizes the chance of guessing correctly. The way to do this is to use the process of elimination. Before you guess, try to eliminate one or more of the answer choices. That way, you can make an educated one out of two or one out of three guess, which is better than one out of four!

Go with Your Gut

In those cases where you are not 100 percent sure of the answer you are choosing, it is often best to go with your gut feeling and stick with your first answer. If you decide to change that answer and pick another one, you may well pick the wrong answer because you have over-thought the problem. More often than not, if you know something about the subject, your first answer is likely to be the correct one.

Be Wary of Answer Choices That Look Familiar but Are Not Correct

Sometimes in the set of answer choices there will be one or more wrong answers that include familiar expressions or phrases. You might be tempted to pick one of these choices if you are working quickly or not paying complete attention. That is why it is important to think through each question thoroughly and carefully to make sure that you pick the correct answer choice.

TIPS FOR TEST DAY

Stay Calm

Once test day comes, you are as prepared as you are ever going to be, so there is no point in panicking. Use your energy to make sure that you are extra careful in answering questions and marking your answer choices.

Watch the Time

Make sure that you are on track to answer all of the questions within the time allowed. With so many questions to answer in a short time period, you are not going to have a lot of time to spare. Check yourself at 10- or 15-minute intervals using your watch or timer. Do not spend too much time on any one question. If you find yourself stuck for more than a minute or two on a question, you should move on.

Do Not Panic If Time Runs Out

If you pace yourself and keep track of your progress, you should not run out of time. If you do, however, do not panic. Because there is no guessing penalty and you have nothing to lose by doing so, enter answers to all the remaining questions. If you are able to make educated guesses, you will probably be able to improve your score. However, even random guesses may help you pick up a few points. Guessing well is a skill that comes with practice, so incorporate it into your preparation program.

Use Extra Time to Check Your Work

If you have time left over at the end of the test, go back and check your work. Make sure that you have marked your answer sheet correctly. Check any calculations you may have made to make sure that they are correct. Resist the urge to second-guess too many of your answers, however, because this may lead you to change an already correct answer to a wrong one.

McGraw-Hill Education

5 NLN PAX-RN

PRACTICE TESTS

Practice Test 1

Verbal Ability
Word Knowledge and Reading Comprehension

45 minutes

WORD KNOWLEDGE: Read each sentence carefully. Then, on the basis of what is stated in the sentence, select the answer to the incomplete statement. The answers will be found at the end of the test.

1. Accepted modes of behavior within a social set are called
   a. orientation.
   b. commemoration.
   c. protégé.
   d. etiquette.

2. Our staff is hoping to emulate the same methods that have brought success to other hospitals around the country.
   Emulate means to
   a. study.
   b. publicize.
   c. imitate.
   d. understand.

3. A person who is denied any contact by his or her own family has been
   a. ostracized.
   b. lauded.
   c. demoted.
   d. promulgated.

4. His opinion of how to treat measles was the exact antithesis of mine.
   Antithesis means
   a. opposite.
   b. opinion.
   c. equivalent.
   d. philosophy.

5. When you meet friends at a rendezvous, you meet
   a. where you live.
   b. outside, not inside.
   c. where you find them.
   d. at an agreed-upon spot.

6. After the hurricane, the house could still be lived in. The house was
   a. repairable.
   b. habitable.
   c. decimated.
   d. delineated.

7. It was a fortuitous turn of events that led Jennifer to our house.
   Fortuitous means
   a. disastrous.
   b. complicated.
   c. lucky.
   d. famous.

8. The only way to remove that dried, crusty glue was with a chemical
   a. solvent.
   b. adhesive.
   c. adherent.
   d. placation.

9. The negative lab results clearly showed that the growth on her arm was completely benign.
   Benign means
   a. unfamiliar.
   b. foreign.
   c. typical.
   d. harmless.

10. If you have an affinity for singing, you are a(n)
    a. expert.
    b. natural.
    c. menace.
    d. fan.

11. A dog trotted aimlessly up and down the beach. The dog was
    a. meandering.
    b. investigating.
    c. disheveled.
    d. contravening.

12. Someone who is both curt and abrupt in manner can be described as
    a. incisive.
    b. brusque.
    c. obsequious.
    d. understated.

13. A solemn compact between two parties could be called a
    a. covenant.
    b. prevarication.
    c. sacrament.
    d. missive.

14. Someone or something that indicates forthcoming bad news is called a
    a. debacle.
    b. harbinger.
    c. fetish.
    d. iconoclast.

15. Although she apologized, the pain she had caused with her words was irrevocable.
    Irrevocable means
    a. permanent.
    b. repairable.
    c. compliant.
    d. accidental.

16. A group of words that doesn't really mean what the words mean is called
    a. an idiom.
    b. a facsimile.
    c. a quibbling.
    d. an extrapolation.

READING COMPREHENSION: There are five reading passages in this section. Read each passage carefully. Then, on the basis of what you have read in the passage, select the best answer for each question.

PASSAGE 1

It is hard to imagine that the virus that causes children to break out into itchy red dots and miss a few days of school is the same one that can send adults to the hospital begging for pain relief, but it is true. The varicella-zoster virus is responsible for both chickenpox in children and shingles in adults. Unlike many other viruses, this herpes virus can hibernate within the body for decades, only becoming noticeable when a person's immune system is severely compromised.

Shingles is often considered one of the most uncomfortable conditions because it causes burning and/or shooting pain, tingling and itching, and commonly rashes or blisters. Treatment ranges from a vaccine that prevents the virus from attacking in the first place to antiviral and pain medications for people who are already affected.

Every year almost one million Americans seek help from the pain and discomfort of shingles, costing the United States $556 million in treatment. Unfortunately, a great many of these victims are also members of a very vulnerable population: the elderly. According to research, people 65 years of age or older are seven times more likely to develop shingles than younger people.

17. What is the main idea of this passage?
    a. The varicella-zoster virus causes both chickenpox and shingles.
    b. Shingles causes people a lot of pain and costs the medical system millions.
    c. The elderly are the age group most at risk for contracting shingles.
    d. A case of chickenpox can often cause children to miss several days of school.

18. Shingles causes all of the following symptoms *except*
    a. pain.
    b. blisters.
    c. fever.
    d. itching.

19. Why is the vaccine the most effective type of treatment?
    a. It is less expensive than the other available options.
    b. It takes effect faster than antiviral and pain medications.
    c. It is particularly effective with the elderly age group.
    d. It prevents the condition from occurring in the first place.

20. Shingles tends to manifest in adults when
    a. their immune system is compromised.
    b. they are just past puberty.
    c. the vaccine is administered.
    d. they are younger than 65 years of age.

21. What makes this virus unusual?
    a. It affects people of all ages.
    b. It often attacks the elderly.
    c. It causes some discomfort.
    d. It can stay dormant for years.

22. The author of this passage would probably support
    a. an increase in the cost of treatment.
    b. a program of vaccination against the virus.
    c. a concentration on the treatment for children.
    d. a decrease in the cost of treatment.

PASSAGE 2

In recent years, there have been frightening headlines about harmful ingredients, such as mercury and lead, in ordinary cosmetics. However, these are hardly the first examples of people paying a heavy price to conform to cultural ideals of beauty. That is a tradition that has been around for centuries.

Ancient Egyptians decorated their eyes with malachite (a green ore of copper), galena (a lead sulfide), and kohl (a paste made from soot, fat, and metals such as lead). This may have made them look more beautiful, but it also led to such health problems as insomnia and mental confusion.

The ancient Greeks went even further. They applied lead to their entire faces, supposedly to clear their complexions of any blemishes and improve the color of their skin. Health problems that resulted ranged from infertility to insanity. The lead ointment whitened their faces—considered a sign of purity—so they then added some red lead to their cheeks for that rosy glow. As if these toxic elements were not enough, they also used hair dyes that contained lead. Some historians suspect that because the Romans favored the same cosmetics as the Greeks did, lead poisoning was part of what later led to the fall of the Roman Empire.

Lead played a huge role in cosmetics for centuries, but it was not until the midnineteenth century that the American Medical Association (AMA) published a paper about the connection between lead in cosmetics and health concerns. Despite the availability of this information, sellers still offered powders and potions that contained harmful chemicals and other materials. These products had such innocuous names as Snow White Enamel, Milk of Roses, and Berry's Freckle Ointment.

The Pure Food and Drug Act (1906) and the creation of the Food and Drug Administration (FDA) helped put an end to some of the most dangerous cosmetics, although products such as a lotion containing rat poison and a mascara that caused blindness still made it onto the market. In 1938, cosmetics came under the control of the FDA, and in 1977, a law was passed requiring cosmetic manufacturers to list all ingredients on their product labels.

Although these steps have helped ensure product safety, problems still exist. As recently as 2007, lipsticks for sale were found to contain lead, and mascara was found to contain mercury. An additional concern is phthalates, industrial chemicals that can cause birth defects and infertility. They are found in personal care products, such as shampoos, lotions, perfume, and deodorants.

An old saying states that beauty has a price. Sometime it just may be higher than consumers realize.

23. Which of these topics is the main focus of the passage?
    a. Frightening news stories from the past
    b. Ancient Egyptian and Greek cultures
    c. The danger of cosmetics throughout history
    d. The control of makeup by the FDA

24. Why did the ancient Greeks put white lead ointment on their faces?
    a. To make themselves look younger.
    b. To clear up their complexions.
    c. To keep from getting seriously ill.
    d. To achieve an overall rosy glow.

25. One might infer from this passage that
    a. For many people, beauty is more important than health.
    b. Manufacturers of cosmetics will continue to ignore FDA rulings.
    c. The AMA regulates cosmetic ingredients.
    d. Phthalates are not nearly as dangerous as ingredients used in the past.

26. Which of the following is identified in the passage as a health hazard resulting from lead?
    a. Cancer
    b. Paralysis
    c. Infertility
    d. Deafness

27. Which of the following types of cosmetics was not mentioned as containing toxic materials?
    a. Lipstick
    b. Deodorant
    c. Mascara
    d. Blush

28. What conclusion can be drawn from the fact that, as recently as 2007, cosmetics were being pulled from store shelves?
    a. The FDA is no longer performing its job properly.
    b. The AMA believes that all cosmetics are completely safe now.
    c. Manufacturers are still using harmful ingredients in their products.
    d. Personal care products that contain phthalates are also being removed from stores.

PASSAGE 3

In some schools around the country, physical education classes look a lot different than they did a generation or two ago. Kids are still in motion, stretching, running, lifting, and sweating. But instead of everyone doing the same activity at the same time as a team, they are exercising independently. They are being taught movements and activities that their teachers hope they will incorporate into their lives rather than just perform long enough to get a good grade.

By teaching kids the pleasure of exercise, gym teachers hope to instill important lessons about maintaining good health, staying fit, and keeping weight under control. By getting the chance to work at their own pace, rather than being forced to keep up with other classmates, students are often more willing to try new things and stick with them. They can also participate in low-impact sports like yoga, martial arts, and weight lifting. Instead of playing basketball or baseball, they can focus on more general skills like passing the ball.

A growing number of physical education (PE) teachers are also putting more of an emphasis on general nutrition and health. According to Craig Buschner, president of the National Association for Sport and Physical Education, "This field has to make changes." With the continual increase in the number of children who are obese, there is greater pressure to teach students about how to stay fit. To do this, gym teachers have to look at new ways to introduce exercise to their classes that will not intimidate or overwhelm them but instead intrigue and engage them.

One other difference found in some modern gym classes is the grading system. Instead of being graded on the ability to run laps in a set time or make a certain number of baskets, the students are graded simply on the effort they make in the class. Some even get extra credit if they are the sweatiest student in the room!

29. What would be the best title for this passage?
    a. Being a Team in PE
    b. A New Kind of Grade
    c. Learning Martial Arts
    d. PE for School and Life

30. The term **instill** as used in the second paragraph of the passage can best be defined as
    a. encourage.
    b. brainwash.
    c. demand.
    d. create.

31. What can you conclude is the primary difference between traditional PE and how some PE classes are being taught today?
    a. For the first time, low-impact sports have been introduced.
    b. Today's students are stretching, running, and lifting.
    c. There is a greater emphasis on lifelong fitness.
    d. Gym teachers are grading more harshly.

32. What can be inferred about the "sweatiest student" referred to in the last sentence of the passage?
    a. This student is more overweight than anyone else.
    b. This student has worked hardest during class.
    c. This student does not need extra credit.
    d. This student is behind all of his/her classmates.

33. According to the passage, PE teachers are trying to teach students lessons about all of the following *except*
    a. the importance of good nutrition for health.
    b. staying generally physically fit.
    c. ways to avoid contracting contagious diseases.
    d. keeping weight under control.

34. Why does the author quote Craig Buschner in the passage?
    a. To make an entirely new point about physical education
    b. To lend authority to ideas presented in the passage
    c. To demonstrate that not all PE teachers are in agreement
    d. To debunk the idea that childhood obesity is a growing problem

PASSAGE 4

According to Professor John MacKinnon, certain places are more likely than others to house new or rediscovered species. First, scientists should look in areas that are geologically stable. Areas with regular earthquakes or volcanic eruptions are less likely to contain species that go back thousands of years, because frequent upheavals are not conducive to steady population growth or a comfortable way of life. Second, scientists are most likely to find undiscovered or rediscovered species in remote, isolated areas. Often, cultivation eliminates the trees or shrubs that house and protect animal life. Third, a stable climate is another thing to look for. Stability of climate ensures that the animals that live in the region have had no reason to leave it in search of warmer or wetter environments.

A fourth key thing scientists should look for, according to MacKinnon, is an area with a variety of unusual species that are specific to that area. Of course, this requirement refers back to requirement number two, isolation. An area that is very isolated or difficult to access will naturally have species that cannot be found anywhere else.

In 1994, American biologist Peter Zahler took his second trip to the isolated valleys of the Diamer region in northern Pakistan. He was searching for the woolly flying squirrel, a dog-sized squirrel last seen in 1924. Working with a guide, Zahler moved from valley to valley. He quizzed the local residents about the squirrel. Many recalled hearing tales about the strange animal, but all insisted that it was extinct.

One day, two men entered Zahler's camp. After some small talk, one asked whether he would be willing to pay for a live squirrel. Zahler agreed to pay top dollar, never envisioning that two hours later, he would be presented with a woolly flying squirrel in a bag. Following that surprise, Zahler located evidence of live squirrels throughout the region. The squirrel certainly met all of MacKinnon's requirements. Despite frequent avalanches, the Himalayas are a geologically stable area with a harsh but stable climate and a number of rare species. Not only were the squirrels' caves remote and isolated, it was often necessary to rappel down or climb up sheer cliffs to reach them.

35. According to the passage, all of these statements are true *except*
    a. "Woolly flying squirrels are larger than most squirrels."
    b. "The Himalayas contain a variety of unique species."
    c. "Animals in a drought may leave for a wetter habitat."
    d. "The woolly flying squirrel was extinct for many years."

36. Which of these would be the **best** title for the passage?
    a. Subtropical Find
    b. Rediscovering Our Planet
    c. Squirrel Supports a Theory
    d. The Animals of Pakistan

37. The author includes the story of the woolly flying squirrel to
    a. provide an example that supports McKinnon's premise.
    b. demonstrate that new species are not always new.
    c. refute McKinnon's notion that climate matters to rediscovery.
    d. contrast one recent rediscovery with another.

38. According to the article, one reason new or long-lost species may be found in areas with stable climates is that
    a. stable climates are often found in areas that are difficult to access.
    b. an unstable climate can decimate an animal population.
    c. without a stable climate, animals may need to migrate or leave.
    d. stable climates appear in regions with geological stability.

39. How is the information in the third paragraph organized?
    a. By reasons and examples
    b. Using comparisons and contrasts
    c. In chronological order
    d. Using cause-and-effect relationships

40. Which of the following statements from the passage provides the least support for the author's claim that Zahler's rediscovery met McKinnon's requirements?
    a. "Despite frequent avalanches, the Himalayas are a geologically stable area with a harsh but stable climate and a number of rare species."
    b. "In 1994, American biologist Peter Zahler took his second trip to the isolated valleys of the Diamer region in northern Pakistan."
    c. "Not only were the squirrels' caves remote and isolated, it was often necessary to rappel down or climb up sheer cliffs to reach them."
    d. "Zahler agreed to pay top dollar, never envisioning that two hours later, he would be presented with a woolly flying squirrel in a bag."

PASSAGE 5

The discovery of electrons came about in a roundabout way. In the latter part of the nineteenth century, a popular demonstration by lecturers involved the cathode ray.

They would evacuate air from a glass tube, pass high voltage through it, and show audiences the patterns of light that appeared. Were these really waves traveling through "ether"? Heinrich Hertz and Phillip Lenard conducted experiments that made this seem possible. On the other hand, English physicists had long posited that there must be a fundamental unit of electricity, a particle that connected matter and electricity. The Irish physicist George Johnstone-Stoney had even gone so far as to calculate its size and to name it *electron*.

French physicist Jean Perrin determined that the cathode rays had negative charges. But it was not until English physicist J. J. Thomson designed an elegant set of experiments that the electron's existence was proved.

The first experiment determined that the negative charge of cathode rays could not be separated from the rays themselves using magnetism. The second found that the rays could bend when influenced by an electric field. The third measured the ratio of charge to mass of the rays by comparing the energy they carried and the amount of deflection possible when an electric field was introduced. Thomson discovered that the ratio was enormous, meaning that the rays were either tiny or very highly charged or both.

His conclusions, published in 1897, involved the existence of a subatomic particle with a negative charge. It was not, however, until Thomson's son, George, proved that electrons, although particles, had many of the properties of a wave, that the mysteries of the cathode ray were truly solved.

George Thomson's concept of wave-particle duality, the notion that matter and light have properties of both waves and particles, was critical to the development of quantum mechanics. It was not a particularly new concept, having roots as far back as Isaac Newton's insistence that light was composed of particles, which he called *corpuscles,* the very word J. J. Thomson used to describe the particles of atoms he found in cathode rays.

41. Which of the following examples is presented as evidence that J. J. Thomson's theory about subatomic particles was not new?
    a. The work of George Johnstone-Stoney
    b. The work of George Thomson
    c. The work of Heinrich Hertz
    d. The work of Phillip Lenard

42. Thomson's first experiment indicated that
    a. unlike most rays, cathode rays were negatively charged.
    b. cathode rays could be diverted using electromagnetism.
    c. the ray's negative charge was embedded within the particles.
    d. most subatomic particles are tiny and highly charged.

43. The discussion of corpuscles in the fifth paragraph shows primarily that
    a. people in the 1600s understood the parts of an atom.
    b. Thomson borrowed a term from a much older theory.
    c. atoms and blood cells are linked by similar structures.
    d. Isaac Newton was trained as a medical doctor.

44. The statement in the first paragraph that "the discovery of electrons came about in a roundabout way" indicates that the author believes that
    a. there is more to discover about electrons.
    b. the discovery of electrons did not proceed step-by-step.
    c. electrons could never have been discovered by a single scientist.
    d. scientists ended up at the beginning when they searched for an answer.

45. The *tone* of this passage suggests that the author
    a. considers J. J. Thomson a splendid scientist.
    b. prefers Isaac Newton to more recent scientists.
    c. would like to know more about George Thomson.
    d. believes that English scientists surpass the French.

46. The author's claim that George Thomson's work was critical to quantum mechanics could *best* be supported by the inclusion of
    a. the theories of light proposed by Isaac Newton and Christian Huygens.
    b. experiments showing the results of gravity on light and sound waves.
    c. de Broglie's equation relating wavelength to momentum.
    d. a definition of quantum mechanics that mentions wave-particle duality.

WORD KNOWLEDGE: Read each sentence carefully. Then, on the basis of what is stated in the sentence, select the answer to the incomplete statement. The answers will be found at the end of the test.

47. The doctor abdicated responsibility for her patient after he refused treatment.
    Abdicate means to
    a. reject.
    b. claim.
    c. blame.
    d. investigate.

48. Public opinion began to **oscillate** after the president had both success and failure in his second term, as reflected in polling results that
    a. crystallized.
    b. claimed.
    c. blamed.
    d. fluctuated.

49. The actress's sighs and blushes when the hero entered stage left were supposed to indicate that she was entirely
    a. dissident.
    b. enamored.
    c. laconic.
    d. dejected.

50. Someone who is filled with **lassitude** is
    a. energetic.
    b. determined.
    c. grieving.
    d. exhausted.

51. Some unorthodox treatments are actually rooted in sound medical practice. **Unorthodox** means
    a. nativistic.
    b. traditional.
    c. unconventional.
    d. uncanny.

52. The hospital administrator was fostering a sense of camaraderie among his staff. **Foster** means to
    a. dread.
    b. anticipate.
    c. avoid.
    d. nurture.

53. After being in the spotlight for three decades, the movie star became a recluse. **Recluse** means
    a. hermit.
    b. seminarian.
    c. extrovert.
    d. polygamist.

54. Although I am completely innocent, I was still accused of nefarious behavior. **Nefarious** means
    a. wicked.
    b. bizarre.
    c. unkind.
    d. sarcastic.

55. If you ask a patient, "What was the last thing you **masticated**?" you are actually asking, "What was the last thing you _____?"
    a. did
    b. chewed
    c. wore
    d. drank

56. In order to blend into the crowds at the coliseum, the prince dressed
    a. insensate.
    b. incognito.
    c. inauspiciously.
    d. imbroglio.

57. "There is no room for rancor between employees," said the head nurse.
    Rancor means
    a. laziness.
    b. miscommunication.
    c. resentment.
    d. impatience.

58. She built a gazebo on top of a small knoll in the back of her property.
    Knoll means
    a. peak.
    b. hill.
    c. fjord.
    d. escarpment.

59. I had been trying to placate the angry patients for several hours, but I was not very successful.
    Placate means
    a. inform.
    b. listen.
    c. calm.
    d. inspire.

60. It seemed irrefutable that the patient was repressing his feelings about the assault.
    Irrefutable means
    a. appropriate.
    b. dubious.
    c. undeniable.
    d. inappropriate.

Mathematics

45 Minutes

Work each problem carefully. Use scrap paper to do your calculations. The correct answers will be found at the end of the test.

1. How many fractions could be derived by dividing $\frac{6}{8}$ by even numbers?
   a. 4
   b. 32
   c. 144
   d. An infinite number

2. $(x^4)^5 =$
   a. $-x$
   b. x^9
   c. x^{12}
   d. x^{20}

3. Express the ratio of 15:40 as a percentage.
   a. 15 percent
   b. 37.5 percent
   c. 62.5 percent
   d. 67.5 percent

4. Maria is three years younger than half the age of one of her regular patients, Dennis. If M is Maria's age and D is Dennis's age, which of the following mathematical statements reflects this relationship?
   a. $M = 2D + 3$
   b. $M = 2D - 3$
   c. $M = \frac{1}{2}D + 3$
   d. $M = \frac{1}{2}D - 3$

5. If someone in a foreign country saw an international broadcast of an American cable news channel weather report that said it was 90°F in Miami, what approximate temperature on the Celsius scale would that viewer understand this to be?
   a. 18°C
   b. 32°C
   c. 48°C
   d. 64°C

6. What is the probability that two cards drawn from a deck of cards are face cards (king, queen, or jack) of any suit if the first card drawn is replaced before the second card is drawn?

    a. $\dfrac{9}{169}$

    b. $\dfrac{1}{16}$

    c. $\dfrac{3}{13}$

    d. $\dfrac{1}{26}$

7. Which of the following numbers is the smallest?
    a. 0.205
    b. 1.1
    c. 0.084
    d. 0.7

8. $385 \div 7 =$
    a. 22
    b. 35
    c. 55
    d. 62

9. $7,236 + 5,971 =$
    a. 10,327
    b. 12,097
    c. 13,207
    d. 14,017

10. Gail owns a flower shop and has decided that as a special promotion, she will make each \$15 arrangement one dollar more than half price. If x is the sale price of one of these arrangements, which of the following mathematical statements represents this best?

    a. $x = \dfrac{1}{2} \times 15 - 1$

    b. $x = \dfrac{1}{2} \times 15 + 1$

    c. $x = \dfrac{1}{2} \times 1 + 15$

    d. $x = \dfrac{1}{2} \times 1 \times 15$

11. A teacher gave a math exam to 15 students. The scores were 94, 71, 68, 83, 80, 86, 76, 86, 91, 97, 88, 77, 85, 70, 78. What is the mean of the data set of grades?
    a. 55
    b. 66
    c. 78
    d. 82

12. Referring to the test scores in question 11, what is the median of the data set of grades?
    a. 80
    b. 83
    c. 85
    d. 86

13. Which of these integers is the largest?
    a. −8
    b. −21
    c. −13
    d. −167

14. A parking lot holds three black cars and two white cars. If the percentages of black and white cars are represented on a pie chart, what is the degree measure of the central angle that represents the black cars?
    a. 60°
    b. 124°
    c. 144°
    d. 216°

15. A package of six cookies is split between two children at snack time. How many cookies does it take to feed 12 children?
    a. 6
    b. 12
    c. 18
    d. 36

16. $593 \div 5 =$
    a. 118 r3
    b. 118 r6
    c. 121 r3
    d. 121 r6

17. How many runners did not finish the race if 40 percent of 250 contestants made it to the end?
    a. 115
    b. 100
    c. 150
    d. 210

Use the following graph for questions 18 and 19.

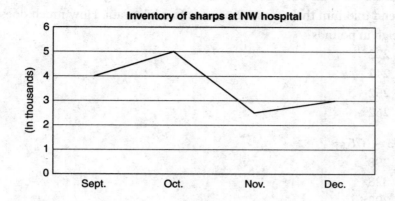

18. Which of the following is the best approximation of the percent decrease in sharps inventory from October to November?
    a. 25
    b. 50
    c. 75
    d. 100

19. If 500 sharps were discarded between the inventory counts in September and October, approximately how many were purchased in the same time period?
    a. 500
    b. 1,000
    c. 1,500
    d. 2,500

20. A certain number is three less than the product of 2 and 10. What is the value of that number?
    a. 10
    b. 17
    c. 20
    d. 23

21. $3.4 \div 0.2 =$
    a. 0.17
    b. 1.7
    c. 17
    d. 170

22. Solve for x: $10 + 5x^2 = 135$
    a. ± 2
    b. ± 5
    c. ± 10
    d. ± 25

23. While visiting another country, Kurt weighed himself on a metric scale. It told him he weighed 110 kilograms. He thought he had lost a lot of weight until a friend told him there was 2.2 pounds to a kilogram. How much does Kurt really weigh in pounds?
    a. 222
    b. 242
    c. 252
    d. 262

24. $673 - 375 =$
    a. 298
    b. 328
    c. 398
    d. 438

25. $782 \times 21 =$
    a. 9,384
    b. 15,640
    c. 16,422
    d. 17,204

26. Solve for x: $4(2x + 20) + 3(x - 1) = 0$
    a. 11
    b. 7
    c. -7
    d. -11

27. If $5y > 6$, y would have to be greater than
    a. 2
    b. 1
    c. -1
    d. $1\frac{1}{5}$

28. Which of the following is the smallest?
    a. $|-3|$
    b. -3
    c. $\frac{1}{3}$
    d. $-\frac{1}{3}$

29. $3,498 \div 26 =$
    a. 105 r6
    b. 134 r14
    c. 215 r12
    d. 232 r12

30. $\dfrac{7}{9} - \dfrac{1}{4} =$

    a. $\dfrac{19}{36}$

    b. $\dfrac{3}{4}$

    c. $\dfrac{37}{36}$

    d. $\dfrac{5}{4}$

31. Which of the following lists is in order from smallest to largest?

    a. $\dfrac{1}{8}, \dfrac{2}{5}, \dfrac{1}{2}, \dfrac{3}{4}$

    b. $\dfrac{2}{5}, \dfrac{1}{8}, \dfrac{3}{4}, \dfrac{1}{2}$

    c. $\dfrac{3}{4}, \dfrac{1}{2}, \dfrac{2}{5}, \dfrac{1}{8}$

    d. $\dfrac{2}{5}, \dfrac{3}{4}, \dfrac{1}{2}, \dfrac{1}{8}$

32. The mixed number $4\dfrac{5}{7}$ expressed as a fraction is

    a. $\dfrac{5}{7}$

    b. $\dfrac{20}{7}$

    c. $\dfrac{33}{7}$

    d. $\dfrac{45}{7}$

33. A doctor prescribes 200 milligrams of a drug per day for 60 days. How many grams of the drug would this prescription use, given that there are 1,000 milligrams in one gram?
    a. 4
    b. 60
    c. 6
    d. 12

34. If the amount of rainfall in one week was measured in centimeters per day and recorded as 3, 4, 0, 2, 0, 3, 0, what was the mode of the rainfall?
    a. 0
    b. 2
    c. 3
    d. 4

35. What is the sum of the prime factors of 28?
    a. 7
    b. 11
    c. 14
    d. 28

36. $4\dfrac{5}{6} - 2\dfrac{3}{4} =$

    a. $\dfrac{12}{25}$

    b. $\dfrac{25}{12}$

    c. $\dfrac{29}{6}$

    d. $\dfrac{11}{12}$

37. What is the simplest form of 80 percent if written as a fraction?

    a. $\dfrac{5}{6}$

    b. $\dfrac{80}{100}$

    c. $\dfrac{8}{100}$

    d. $\dfrac{8}{10}$

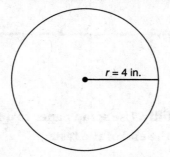

$r = 4$ in.

38. What is the circumference of the preceding circle?
    a. 8 in.
    b. 16 in.
    c. 8π in.
    d. 16π in.

39. What is the median of −8, 12, 3, 4, and −1?
    a. 2
    b. 3
    c. 4
    d. 8

40. $0.38 \times 2.35 =$
    a. 0.273
    b. 0.893
    c. 2.73
    d. 8.93

Science

45 Minutes

Work each problem carefully. Use scrap paper to do your calculations. The correct answers will be found at the end of the test.

1. In classifying all living things on Earth, which of the following groups would sort all life into two groups?
    a. Vertebrates/Invertebrates
    b. Mammals/Birds
    c. Prokaryotes/Eukaryotes
    d. Protista/Fungi

2. Given one mole of O_2 gas at STP, what is the mass of this sample?
    a. 8 grams
    b. 16 grams
    c. 32 grams
    d. 64 grams

3. Which of the following is not a type of muscle?
    a. Nervous muscle
    b. Smooth muscle
    c. Skeletal muscle
    d. Cardiac muscle

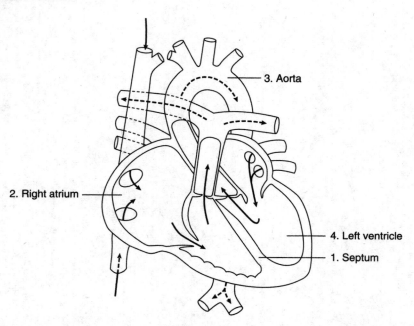

3. Aorta

2. Right atrium

4. Left ventricle

1. Septum

4. As shown in the heart diagram on the previous page, separating the left and right sides of the heart is the
   a. 1.
   b. 2.
   c. 3.
   d. 4.

5. Animals like snails and clams contained within a hard shell differ from humans because they lack
   a. bones.
   b. nerves.
   c. appendages.
   d. shells.

6. Quantities having both magnitude and direction are
   a. scalar quantities.
   b. vector quantities.
   c. directional quantities.
   d. matrices.

7. The arrow in the following diagram represents the wave's

   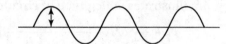

   a. period.
   b. frequency.
   c. amplitude.
   d. wavelength.

8. Exactly 2.0 moles of an element weigh 8.0 grams. Which of the following is true?
   a. One mole of the element weighs 16.0 grams, and the element is sulfur, S.
   b. The element in question is beryllium, Be.
   c. One mole of the element also weighs 8.0 grams, and the element is oxygen, O.
   d. One mole of the element weighs 4.0 grams, and the element is helium, He.

9. The heart is composed of which type of tissue?
   a. Cardiac muscle
   b. Ligaments
   c. Smooth tendons
   d. Cartilage

10. A secondary defense for the body against pathogens is
    a. tears.
    b. urine.
    c. inflammation.
    d. mucus.

11. What is the temperature as shown on this thermometer?

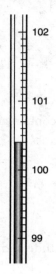

a. 98.5
b. 100.4
c. 100.8
d. 101.4

12. The following diagram illustrates which type of circuit?

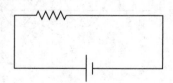

a. Series
b. Parallel
c. Complex
d. Open

13. Given 3.0 moles of krypton gas, Kr(g), how many liters will this sample occupy at STP?
a. 11.2
b. 22.4
c. 44.8
d. 67.2

14. The growth and development of bone is assisted by the use of vitamin D because vitamin D can
a. help the body excrete excess salt.
b. control sulfur and calcium levels in the blood.
c. aid in the absorption of calcium.
d. regulate levels of chloride ion.

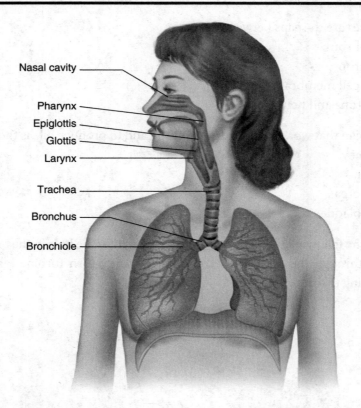

15. The larynx is covered by the _____ so that food does not enter the trachea.
    a. esophagus
    b. pharynx
    c. bronchus
    d. epiglottis

16. The function of the diaphragm in a human being is
    a. to assist the process of respiration.
    b. to conduct the flow of lymph.
    c. to provide structure and protection of organs.
    d. to allow development of a fertilized egg.

17. In a sound wave with a constant velocity, the frequency is inversely proportional
    to the
    a. amplitude.
    b. reflection.
    c. wavelength.
    d. resonance.

18. What is the percent of oxygen in H_2O?
    a. 11.1
    b. 33.3
    c. 88.98
    d. 100.0

19. Synapses are the gaps between
    a. nephrons.
    b. neurons.
    c. the cell membrane.
    d. protons and neutrons.

20. The organ that works to detoxify the blood and to produce bile is the
    a. kidney.
    b. liver.
    c. pancreas.
    d. gallbladder.

21. Study the following wave power device. Waves enter the hole in the break wall and travel through the tube. How could it constantly turn turbine blades without damaging them?

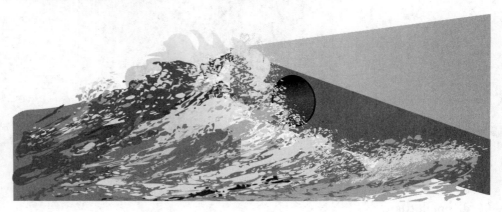

    a. By striking the back of the tube
    b. By forcing air through a pipe
    c. By drawing air back through a pipe
    d. By forcing air in and out through a pipe

22. Force multiplied by distance equals
    a. joules.
    b. work.
    c. power.
    d. potential energy.

23. Given a sample of $C_6H_{12}O_6$(aq), which of the following is true?
    a. The glucose is the solvent and water is the solute.
    b. The glucose is the solvent and water is the solvent.
    c. The glucose is the solute and water is the solute.
    d. The glucose is the solute and water is the solvent.

24. The small intestine contains a large quantity of villi that help
    a. absorb acids and saliva from the mouth.
    b. provide a greater surface for absorption of materials passing through the digestive tract.
    c. produce saliva.
    d. secrete hydrochloric acid to break down foods.

25. Which of the following glands is not paired up with a hormone that it produces?
    a. Testes/Testosterone
    b. Adrenal medulla/Estrogen
    c. Adrenal cortex/Cortisol
    d. Pancreas/Insulin

26. Which of the following causes and effects would occur last in a shallow forest pond that is not fed with a source of freshwater replacement like a larger river?
    a. More consumers in the food chain
    b. A lack of available food
    c. A rapid die-off of mature fish
    d. An increased bloom of algae

27. An object is moving at a constant speed of 12 m/s. That object's acceleration is
    a. 0 k/s^2
    b. 6 m/s^2
    c. 12 m/s^2
    d. 1 m/s^2

28. If 58.5 of NaCl (1 mole of NaCl) are dissolved in enough water to make 0.500 L of solution, what is the molarity of this solution?
    a. 2.0 moles
    b. 11.7 moles
    c. 1.0 moles
    d. The answer cannot be determined from the information given.

29. The process by which oxygen travels from the air into your lungs and then into your blood is called
    a. hypertonic.
    b. osmosis.
    c. diffusion.
    d. passive transport.

30. The brain and the spinal cord make up the
    a. peripheral nervous system.
    b. somatic nervous system.
    c. autonomic nervous system.
    d. central nervous system.

31. Before an object begins its motion it possesses
    a. thermal energy.
    b. potential energy.
    c. kinetic energy.
    d. nuclear energy.

32. A cell is in a solution in which the concentration of solutes is higher inside the cell than outside the cell. The cells will likely
    a. swell up and possibly burst.
    b. shrivel and shrink.
    c. maintain its size.
    d. grow a cell wall for support.

33. A salt solution has a molarity of 1.5 M. How many moles of this salt are present in 2.0 L of this solution?
    a. 1.5 moles
    b. 2.0 moles
    c. 3.0 moles
    d. 0.75 mole

34. Which of the following are considered normal values for the measurements of a person's pulse and blood pressure?
    a. 72 beats per minute and 120 over 80 mm Hg
    b. 100 beats per minute and 140 over 100 mm Hg
    c. 160 beats per minute and 100 over 70 mm Hg
    d. 55 beats per minute and 75 over 60 mm Hg

35. Ligaments hold
    a. bone to bone.
    b. bone to muscle.
    c. tendons to bone.
    d. cartilage to tendons.

36. Avogadro's number is the number of
    a. moles in a sample.
    b. representative elements.
    c. grams in a molecule.
    d. molar masses.

37. A sound wave with a bright timbre is being described by its
    a. loudness.
    b. pitch.
    c. quality.
    d. frequency.

38. Yeast is used to make bread rise because
    a. the yeast engages in photosynthesis, which produces oxygen gas.
    b. carbon dioxide forms while the yeast carries out photosynthesis.
    c. the yeast carries out fermentation, which produces ethanol and carbon dioxide.
    d. yeast breathes in oxygen and produces carbon dioxide as aerobic respiration takes place.

39. Which statement does not have the same truth value as the others?
    a. RNA is single-stranded.
    b. RNA contains uracil.
    c. DNA codes for proteins.
    d. DNA cannot be altered.

40. As water is evaporated from a solution, the concentration of the solute in the solution will
    a. increase.
    b. decrease.
    c. remain the same.
    d. evaporate as well.

41. An atom becomes an ion that possesses a negative charge. The atom must have
    a. gained protons.
    b. lost protons.
    c. lost electrons.
    d. gained electrons.

42. Which substance shows a decrease in solubility in water with an increase in temperature?
    a. NaCl
    b. O_2
    c. KI
    d. $CaCl_2$

43. The retina transmits nerve impulses to the brain via the
    a. optic nerve.
    b. cranial nerve.
    c. cardiac nerve.
    d. esophagus.

44. Which muscle pushes food through the digestive system?
    a. Renal
    b. Smooth
    c. Cardiac
    d. Rough

Characteristics of acid-base disturbances			
Disorder	pH	Primary problem	Compensation
Metabolic acidosis	↓	↓ in HCO_3^-	↓ in $PaCO_2$
Metabolic alkalosis	↑	↑ in HCO_3^-	↑ in $PaCO_2$
Respiratory acidosis	↓	↑ in $PaCO_2$	↑ in $[HCO_3^-]$
Respiratory alkalosis	↑	↓ in $PaCO_2$	↓ in $[HCO_3^-]$

45. According the table above, a patient with an elevated $PaCO_2$ count needs
    a. a decrease in $PaCO_2$ (partial pressure of carbon dioxide) in the blood.
    b. a decrease in HCO_3^- (carbonic acid).
    c. an increase in $PaCO_2$.
    d. an increase in HCO_3^-.

46. Given patients whose age, weight, sex, and temperament are nearly identical, what should the normal values of blood pressure and pulse be during routine examinations and measurements by a physician?
    a. 120/80 mm/Hg and 72/min
    b. 68/116 mm/Hg and 82/min
    c. 102/80 mm/Hg and 62/min
    d. 120/90 mm/Hg and 53/min

47. Which of the following is a way in which mitosis differs from meiosis?
    a. Mitosis takes place to form sex cells.
    b. Meiosis creates cells with half the number of chromosomes of the original cell.
    c. Telophase does not take place in mitosis.
    d. Spermatogenesis and oogenesis occur via mitosis.

48. The ribs are _____ to the lungs in the human body.
    a. medial
    b. distal
    c. anterior
    d. deep

49. Salt is added to a sample of water. Which of the following is true?
    a. The boiling point will increase and the freezing point will decrease.
    b. The boiling point will increase and the freezing point will increase.
    c. The boiling point will decrease and the freezing point will increase.
    d. The boiling point will decrease and the freezing point will decrease.

50. Organic compounds are the basis for life as we know it because
    a. carbon-to-carbon bonds are strong.
    b. carbon can form long chains.
    c. carbon chains can include other elements to give rise to different functional groups.
    d. All of the above.

51. A person gets hit in the face with a puck while playing a game of ice hockey and fractures a bone. Which bone is a most likely candidate for this fracture?
    a. Mandible
    b. Rib
    c. Radius
    d. Femur

52. The word **renal** refers to the
    a. liver.
    b. gallbladder.
    c. kidney.
    d. lung.

53. Which reproductive organ belongs to a different system from the other three?
    a. Follicle
    b. Oviduct
    c. Uterus
    d. Epididymis

54. The iris and retina are parts of the
    a. eye.
    b. ear.
    c. tongue.
    d. skin.

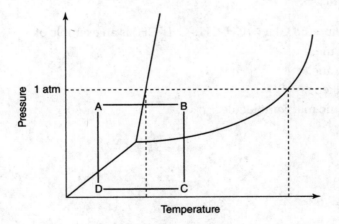

55. Which transition on the phase diagram will include melting?
    a. A→B
    b. B→C
    c. A→D
    d. C→D

56. During breathing, the air pressure in the lungs changes as a result of
    a. constriction of the larynx.
    b. contraction of the diaphragm.
    c. extension of the ribs.
    d. reduction of lung capacity.

57. Which of the following statements is true?
    a. The digestive system can do its job without the use of accessory organs.
    b. The digestive system uses sphincters to contain substances being digested at certain points of the digestive tract.
    c. Mechanical digestion is more important than chemical digestion.
    d. The juices that are used to digest food can be effective at any point along the digestive tract.

58. The heart and veins have valves to ensure that
    a. blood flows in only one direction.
    b. oxygen and carbon dioxide can be exchanged.
    c. lymph can be directed through the arteries.
    d. platelets do not clot at the site of a wound.

59. The name of the compound $CH_3-CH_2-CH_2-CH_3$ is most likely
    a. cyclobutane.
    b. butane.
    c. butene.
    d. butyne.

60. The compound $CH_2 = CH-CH_2-CH_2-CH_3$ is an example of
    a. pentane.
    b. a hexane.
    c. an alkene.
    d. organic macromolecule.

Practice Test 2

Verbal Ability
Word Knowledge and Reading Comprehension

45 minutes

WORD KNOWLEDGE: Read each sentence carefully. Then, on the basis of what is stated in the sentence, select the answer to the incomplete statement. The answers will be found at the end of the test.

1. The _____ patron always gave generously to the hospital's fundraisers.
   a. altruistic
   b. cantankerous
   c. depraved
   d. ethereal

2. Upon returning from their travels, the explorers received both praise and
   a. hiatus.
   b. recompense.
   c. truncheon.
   d. liaison.

3. The survivor told an amazing tale of courage, but many doubters felt it was
   a. cryptic.
   b. indubitable.
   c. bogus.
   d. sentient.

4. Which of the following words is a synonym for the word **homogeneous**?
   a. Assorted
   b. Anonymous
   c. Diverse
   d. Uniform

5. The new head nurse was extremely meticulous and made us double-check every entry in our reports.
   Meticulous means
   a. irresponsible.
   b. careful.
   c. punctual.
   d. knowledgeable.

6. If a doctor informs you that the patient has a **vascular** problem, that means the patient has a condition involving the
   a. reproductive system.
   b. nervous system.
   c. circulatory system.
   d. digestive system.

7. A patient told you that the pain comes and goes in no recognized pattern. Which of the following words would you put into your notes to indicate this?
   a. Acute
   b. Sporadic
   c. Chronic
   d. Consistent

8. The shy new intern spoke with great temerity.
   Temerity means
   a. audacity.
   b. reticence.
   c. embarrassment.
   d. resourcefulness.

9. The king felt his knights were loyal, but it turned out that they were
   a. perfidious.
   b. sedentary.
   c. lugubrious.
   d. sublime.

10. The physician was determined to extricate the splinter, but the task was proving difficult.
    Extricate means
    a. replace.
    b. bandage.
    c. remove.
    d. soften.

11. Although I appreciate your _____, I don't agree with your opinion on the matter at all.
    a. amity
    b. candor
    c. flippancy
    d. repugnance

12. Draining a swollen join can alleviate pressure.
    Alleviate means
    a. lessen.
    b. magnify.
    c. substitute.
    d. vaporize.

13. He paused in his climb up the precipice in a potentially unstable position. It seemed
    a. indomitable.
    b. unbowing.
    c. inflexible.
    d. precarious.

14. A proper formal letter always begins with a salutation.
    A **salutation** is a
    a. commendation.
    b. postscript.
    c. greeting.
    d. signature.

15. Someone within a community who is shunned by the members is called a
    a. sycophant.
    b. defendant.
    c. pariah.
    d. parasite.

16. As they learn more, some students may begin to dispute their teachers.
    Dispute means
    a. approximate.
    b. outpace.
    c. deconstruct.
    d. contradict.

READING COMPREHENSION: There are five reading passages in this section. Read each passage carefully. Then, on the basis of what you have read in the passage, select the best answer for each question.

PASSAGE 1

Most people get a little grumpy when they do not get enough sleep, but when it comes to children, the problem may be more than just some extra irritation. Lack of sleep may also affect their weight, as well as their overall behavior.

A study conducted in New Zealand at the University of Auckland and published in the medical journal *Sleep* followed almost 600 children from infancy through seven years of age. Researchers observed the children's sleep patterns and found that generally they slept less on the weekends than during the week and even less during the summer months.

According to the findings, the children who tended to sleep the least were at greater risk for being overweight and/or experiencing behavioral problems. In fact, those who regularly slept less than 9 hours a night were three times more likely than longer sleepers to be obese and to show signs of attention deficit disorder (ADD) and attention deficit hyperactivity disorder (ADHD). These results were based on questionnaires handed out to the children's parents and teachers.

How does sleep affect weight? The answer to that is still not clear, but experts suspect that chronic sleep deprivation somehow alters the hormones involved in appetite control and metabolism. This is a connection that still needs to be explored to be better understood.

How much sleep is enough for a child? Experts recommend that preschoolers get 11 to 13 hours of sleep each night, whereas school-age children should get between 10 and 11 hours per night. Many children average only 8 hours.

The study concluded that sleep duration is one risk factor that can be fairly easily altered to prevent future health problems for today's young people.

17. What would be the best title for this passage?
    a. Preventing ADHD in Your Child
    b. The Cure for Childhood Obesity
    c. Hormones and Appetite Control
    d. Children and the Need for Sleep

18. This passage suggests that children sleep the most during the
    a. week.
    b. weekend.
    c. summer.
    d. holidays.

19. This study was conducted primarily through
    a. lab experiments.
    b. questionnaires.
    c. brief research.
    d. years of interviews.

20. According to the passage, inadequate sleep can result in all of the following *except*
    a. hyperactivity.
    b. obesity.
    c. irritability.
    d. anorexia.

21. What conclusion can you draw about the connection between sleep and young children?
    a. Lack of sleep causes children to fail in school.
    b. Inadequate rest raises the risk of behavioral and physical problems.
    c. Sleeping less than 10 hours a night is guaranteed to result in obesity.
    d. Eight hours of sleep each night meets the requirement of most children.

22. According to the passage, which of the following ideas needs further exploration?
    a. How much sleep children actually need at each age
    b. How children's sleep patterns change during the seasons
    c. How sleep affects children's appetite and overall metabolism
    d. How teachers and physicians determine a diagnosis of ADD or ADHD

PASSAGE 2

The use of inhaled anesthetics can be traced back as far as the medieval Moors, who used narcotic-soaked sponges placed over the nostrils of patients. Some 300 years later, in 1275, Majorcan alchemist Raymundus Lullus is supposed to have discovered the chemical compound later called ether. The compound which would later have a brief but important run as the anesthetic of choice in Western medicine was synthesized by German physician Valerius Cordus in 1540. Adding sulfuric acid, known at the time as "oil of vitriol," to ethyl alcohol resulted in the compound Cordus called "sweet vitriol."

During the next few centuries, ether was used by physicians for a variety of purposes. Its effectiveness as a hypnotic agent was well known, and a favorite pastime of medical students in the early nineteenth century was the "ether frolic," an early version of the drunken frat party. Nevertheless, no record of ether's being used as an anesthetic in surgery appears until the 1840s.

Dr. Crawford Williamson Long of Jefferson, Georgia, removed neck tumors from a patient under ether anesthesia on March 30, 1842. However, he failed to publish the record of his experiment until 1848, by which time Dr. William T. G. Morton, a dentist in Hartford, Connecticut, had conducted a variety of experiments with ether on animals and himself, culminating in the painless extraction of a tooth from a patient under ether on September 30, 1846.

After reading about Morton's successful use of ether, doctors at Harvard invited him to demonstrate his technique. At Massachusetts General Hospital on October 16, 1846, Morton administered ether to a patient, and a senior surgeon, John Collins Warren, removed a growth from the patient's neck as a crowd of doctors and dignitaries looked on. The operation is recorded in several paintings of the era, indicating its critical importance. Despite its volatility and side effects, ether continued to be used as an anesthetic until it was overtaken by less harmful potions. Morton, meanwhile, struggled unsuccessfully to be granted a patent for his "discovery" and then, when that failed, for his "technique." After years of litigation, he died penniless at age 49.

23. The statement in the first paragraph that ether would "have a brief but important run as the anesthetic of choice in Western medicine" implies that the author believes that
    a. ether was not a particularly good anesthetic.
    b. ether was not used long enough to judge its effectiveness.
    c. ether was effective during the period when it was used.
    d. ether was a noteworthy import from the East to the West.

24. Which of these would be the *best* title for the passage?
    a. Inhaled Anesthetics
    b. An Important Anesthetic
    c. How Anesthetics Have Changed
    d. Our Debt to Ancient Physicians

25. Which of the following statements from the passage provides the least support for the author's claim that ether was an important discovery for physicians at the time?
    a. "Dr. Crawford Williamson Long of Jefferson, Georgia, removed neck tumors from a patient under ether anesthesia on March 30, 1842."
    b. "After reading about Morton's successful use of ether, doctors at Harvard invited him to demonstrate his technique."
    c. "The operation is recorded in several paintings of the era, indicating its critical importance."
    d. "Nevertheless, no record of ether's being used as an anesthetic in surgery appears until the 1840s."

26. In the first paragraph, the author probably writes that Lullus "is supposed to have discovered" ether because
    a. there is conflicting evidence about his discovery.
    b. Lullus did not really discover ether at all.
    c. although Lullus was meant to discover it, someone else did.
    d. no one can really "discover" a chemical compound.

27. How is the information in the fourth paragraph organized?
    a. By reasons and examples
    b. Using comparisons and contrasts
    c. In time order
    d. Using cause-and-effect relationships

28. The author probably includes information about Dr. Long in the third paragraph to show that
    a. Morton was not the first to use ether in a surgical procedure.
    b. publishing results can mean the difference between fortune and penury.
    c. both dentists and doctors used ether to good effect.
    d. doctors in the Northeast often received more attention than Southern doctors.

PASSAGE 3

Aluminum is the most abundant metallic element in the Earth's crust, but it is never found naturally as an element. Instead, it always appears naturally in its oxidized form as a hydroxide we call bauxite.

The extraction of aluminum from bauxite requires three stages. First, the ore is mined. Then it is refined to recover alumina. Finally, the alumina is smelted to produce aluminum.

The mining is done via the open-cut method. Bulldozers remove the topsoil, and excavators or other types of power machinery are used to remove the underlying layer of bauxite. The bauxite may be washed to remove clay and other detritus.

Refining is done via the Bayer refining process, named after its inventor, Karl Bayer. Ground bauxite is fed into a digester, where it is mixed with a caustic soda. The aluminum oxide reacts with the soda to form a solution of sodium aluminate and a precipitate of sodium aluminum silicate. The solution is separated from the silicate through washing and pumping, and the alumina is precipitated from the solution, where it appears as crystals of alumina hydrate. The crystals are washed again to remove any remaining solution. Then they are heated to remove water, leaving the gritty alumina.

Smelting is done via the Hall-Heroult smelting process. An electric current is passed through a molten solution of alumina and cryolite, which is in a cell lined at the bottom and top with carbon. This forces the oxygen to combine with the carbon at the top of the cell, making carbon dioxide, while the molten metallic aluminum collects at the bottom of the cell, where it is siphoned off, cleaned up, and cast into bars, sheets, or whatever form is needed.

As with all mining of metals, bauxite mining presents certain hazards. Along with the usual mining issues of degraded soil and polluted runoff, chief among them is the omnipresent bauxite dust, which clogs machinery and lungs, sometimes for miles around the mining site. Jamaica and Brazil have seen widespread protests recently against the major bauxite mining companies, which continue to insist that no link between bauxite dust and pervasive lung problems has been proved.

29. In the context of the second paragraph, the word **refined** means
    a. superior.
    b. polished.
    c. processed.
    d. restricted.

30. Based on the information in the third paragraph, you can conclude that bauxite is located
    a. within the topsoil.
    b. wherever clay is found.
    c.. below the topsoil.
    d. below the Earth's crust.

31. All of these are produced by the Bayer process *except*
    a. sodium aluminum silicate.
    b. sodium aluminate.
    c. aluminum manganese.
    d. alumina hydrate.

32. The ideas in the third, fourth, and fifth paragraphs are related because they are
    a. steps in a process.
    b. examples of a mineral.
    c. reasons for mining.
    d. comparisons of theories.

33. The author includes the discussion of protests primarily to show that
    a. bauxite mining takes place in the Third World.
    b. workers are starting to fight back against the dangers of mining.
    c. mining companies have misled people for decades.
    d. the government of Brazil works with the mining companies.

34. The *tone* of the passage suggests that the author would most likely believe that
    a. bauxite mining poses health problems.
    b. the United States should use less aluminum.
    c. Australian bauxite is the best quality.
    d. Karl Bayer was something of a genius.

PASSAGE 4

Over the years, acupuncture has become a more widely accepted type of alternative medicine. It is used for a wide variety of ailments, and if a recent study from Germany is valid, relieving menstrual pain can be added to the continuously growing list.

Traditionally, nonsteroidal anti-inflammatory drugs (NSAIDs) are the typical treatment for menstrual discomfort. However, as many consumers and physicians are aware, NSAIDs have a number of side effects, including nausea, vomiting, rash, dizziness, headache, and drowsiness. Acupuncture rarely has any kind of side effects other than the occasional stinging sensation when the needle is inserted or a deep ache around it after it is in place.

Acupuncture has proven helpful in relieving a number of kinds of pain, so researchers at Charité University Medical Center in Berlin wanted to find out how effective it might be in combating cramps and other menstrual discomforts.

More than 200 women were enrolled in the study, and after three months and approximately 10 sessions, the women who were treated with acupuncture reported significantly less pain than those in the control group who received no treatment at all. They also reported a 33 percent improvement in their symptoms. Because of these findings, the researchers came to the conclusion that "acupuncture should be considered as a viable option in the management of these patients."

35. What is the best title for this passage?
   a. A Miracle Cure for Cramps Discovered
   b. Throw Away the Pills and Bring in the Needles
   c. Acupuncture Holds Promise for Combating Menstrual Pain
   d. Alternative Medicine Tries to Prove Itself Better Than Traditional

36. Why were experts interested in finding an alternative treatment for menstrual discomfort?
   a. The usual treatment may produce a number of side effects.
   b. The usual treatment is not profitable enough.
   c. The usual treatment has repeatedly been proved ineffective.
   d. The usual treatment can be too expensive for some families.

37. Why did experts believe that acupuncture might help with menstrual cramps?
   a. Multiple studies suggested that acupuncture would help.
   b. Acupuncture has been effective in treating other types of pain.
   c. Repeated testimonials from patients convinced them.
   d. Acupuncture is a technique that has been used for hundreds of years.

38. What is the main advantage that acupuncture has over NSAIDs?
   a. It costs less.
   b. It is easier to find.
   c. It carries less risk.
   d. It is more effective.

39. What conclusion is suggested by this study from Germany?
   a. So far, acupuncture does not have much credibility as a treatment option.
   b. Acupuncture can relieve women of all menstrual discomfort.
   c. NSAIDs are generally more effective than acupuncture for treating cramps.
   d. Acupuncture is a reasonable treatment choice for cramps.

40. Which fact from the passage suggests that it is not surprising that acupuncture would be an effective treatment for menstrual pain?
    a. Anti-inflammatory drugs (NSAIDs) are the typical treatment for menstrual discomfort.
    b. Acupuncture has become a more widely accepted type of alternative medicine. It is used for a wide variety of ailments.
    c. More than 200 women were enrolled in the study for three months and approximately 10 sessions.
    d. Acupuncture rarely has any kind of side effects other than the occasional stinging sensation.

PASSAGE 5

If statistics are to be believed, the surgeons on the popular television show *Nip/Tuck* seem to be inspiring many viewers to have cosmetic work done. According to the American Society of Aesthetic Plastic Surgery, 11.7 million cosmetic procedures were performed in the United States in 2007 at an overall cost of approximately $13.2 billion. Since 1997, the number of regular surgical procedures has gone up by 114 percent, but the number of nonsurgical procedures has gone up an amazing 754 percent. The vast majority of cosmetic surgery patients are women, perhaps because in so many circumstances, women are more likely than men to be judged by their appearance.

By far, the most popular cosmetic surgical procedure is liposuction, followed by breast augmentation, eyelid surgery, abdominoplasty (often known as a "tummy tuck"), and breast reduction. Common nonsurgical cosmetic procedures include the extremely popular Botox injections, followed by laser hair removal, microdermabrasion, and laser skin resurfacing.

Although more than 90 percent of the patients who undergo cosmetic procedures are women, the number of men having some kind of work is slowly growing. To date, men's favorite procedure is injections to fill out wrinkles.

41. The best title for this passage is
    a. Watching *Nip/Tuck* Is a Smart Thing to Do.
    b. Cosmetic Procedures Are on the Rise.
    c. Liposuction Remains a Popular Choice.
    d. Men Are Getting Rid of Wrinkles.

42. What can be inferred from the fact that women make up the majority of patients for cosmetic procedures?
    a. Women have more money to spend than men.
    b. Women feel more pressure to look attractive.
    c. Women have done more research on the topic.
    d. Women have more patience for recovery.

43. Which of the following is one of the most popular types of cosmetic procedures for women?
    a. Botox injections
    b. Breast reductions
    c. Microdermabrasion
    d. Breast augmentation

44. Which of the following is one of the most popular types of cosmetic procedures for men?
    a. Liposuction
    b. Eyelid surgery
    c. Wrinkle injections
    d "Tummy tucks"

45. What conclusion can be drawn from the fact that the number of men having cosmetic procedures are increasing?
    a. Men are discovering the many cosmetic procedures that are available.
    b. Men are finding out the psychological benefits of Botox injections.
    c. Men are under more social pressure to maintain a handsome appearance.
    d. Men are figuring out that liposuction can bring health benefits.

46. With the information given in the passage, we may infer that viewers of the television show
    a. are mostly men who want to look younger.
    b. seek out treatment for regular surgical procedures.
    c. find plastic surgeons to consult by watching the show.
    d. appreciate the results of the cosmetic procedures they see.

WORD KNOWLEDGE: Read each sentence carefully. Then, on the basis of what is stated in the sentence, select the answer to the incomplete statement. The answers will be found at the end of the test.

47. Despite a limited amount of training, her bedside manner was excellent. She had a(n) _____ understanding of how a patient would like to be treated.
    a. experienced
    b. intuitive
    c. altruistic
    d. communicative

48. Her decision not to perform the operation was scrutinized by everyone at the hospital.
    Scrutinize means to
    a. examine.
    b. applaud.
    c. criticize
    d. misunderstand.

49. People tried their best to stop the floodwaters from reaching the house, but the outcome was_____.
    a. punctual
    b. unforeseen
    c. malicious
    d. inevitable

50. Which of the following words is a synonym for the word **placid**?
    a. Rancid
    b. Improper
    c. Tranquil
    d. Missing

51. The doctor was predicting that the new policies would engender a feeling of discontent at the office.
    Engender means to
    a. diminish.
    b. generate.
    c. soften.
    d. dampen.

52. The relationship between the president and Congress eroded over time.
    Eroded means
    a. engorged.
    b. rehabilitated.
    c. deteriorated.
    d. enlightened.

53. The young sailors performed admirably despite being
    a. without merit.
    b. under duress.
    c. in absentia.
    d. well trained.

54. The commentators discussed a purported settlement of the strike.
    Purported means
    a. announced.
    b. purposeful.
    c. rebutted.
    d. rumored.

55. We had high hopes of bringing our project to
    a. fruition.
    b. agreement.
    c. simulacrum.
    d. stipend.

56. Which of the following means the opposite of **sagacity**?
    a. Wisdom
    b. Imprudence
    c. Protocol
    d. Stature

57. Which of the following is a synonym for **affinity**?
    a. Kinship
    b. Leadership
    c. Immensity
    d. Variation

58. The new administration keeps telling us that we have to cut costs, so we need to be_____.
    a. impersonal
    b. exuberant
    c. frugal
    d. contrite

59. Harry didn't like haunted house tours because he found them extremely
    a. exotic.
    b. tenuous.
    c. macabre.
    d. petulant.

60. The new hotel was too opulent for my relatives who were simple folk.
    Opulent means
    a. obsolete.
    b. panoramic.
    c. fearful.
    d. lavish.

Mathematics

45 Minutes

Work each problem carefully. Use scrap paper to do your calculations. The correct answers will be found at the end of the test.

1. $(2.4 \times 10^6) \div (-1.2 \times 10^3) =$
    a. -2.0×10^3
    b. -2.0×10^4
    c. 2.0×10^3
    d. 2.0×10^6

2. $3.2 \times 4.16 =$
    a. 13.213
    b. 13.312
    c. 13.320
    d. 13.023

3. Express in scientific notation: 13.9.
    a. 1.39×10^{-1}
    b. 1.39×10^1
    c. 13.9×10^{-1}
    d. 13.9×10^1

4. The ratio of boys to girls in the graduating class of a school is 3:2. If there are a total of 430 students in the class, how many girls are in the graduating class?
    a. 74
    b. 86
    c. 172
    d. 215

5. $(6x^2y^5z^3) \div (3x^2y^3z^6) =$
    a. $\dfrac{z^2}{2y^3}$

    b. $\dfrac{y^2}{2z^3}$

    c. $\dfrac{2y^2}{z^3}$

    d. $\dfrac{2z^2}{y^3}$

6. Solve for x: $\dfrac{x^2 + x - 42}{x + 7} = 1$
    a. −7
    b. 2
    c. 6
    d. 7

7. A package weighing $7\dfrac{2}{3}$ pounds needs to be mailed and the postal rate is 13 cents per pound. What would be the cost rounded to the nearest cent?
    a. $0.13
    b. $0.91
    c. $1.00
    d. $7.62

8. What percent of 920 is 1,104?
    a. 80 percent
    b. 85 percent
    c. 120 percent
    d. 310 percent

9. How many meters are there in 435 centimeters if 1 decimeter equals 10 centimeters and 10 decimeters equal 1 meter?
    a. 43.5
    b. 4.35
    c. 0.435
    d. 435

10. $7 - 3\dfrac{2}{3} =$
    a. $4\dfrac{1}{3}$
    b. $3\dfrac{1}{3}$
    c. $3\dfrac{2}{3}$
    d. $2\dfrac{1}{3}$

11. $38 \times \dfrac{7}{16} =$
    a. 16
    b. 13
    c. $\dfrac{133}{8}$
    d. $\dfrac{266}{38}$

12. For every four family farms in America, only one is profitable. If there are 1,890,000 family farms in the United States, how many are profitable?
    a. 725,000
    b. 7,250,000
    c. 252,000
    d. 472,500

Use the bar graph below for questions 13 and 14.

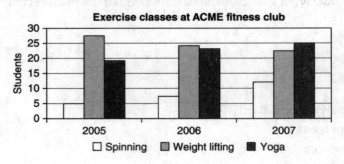

13. Which class or classes have seen participation increase over both years?
    a. Both spinning and yoga
    b. Weight lifting
    c. Yoga
    d. Both spinning and weight lifting

14. Which class has seen the largest change in participation (increase or decrease) from any year to the next?
    a. Spinning
    b. Weight lifting
    c. Yoga
    d. Both spinning and yoga

15. What is the average (mean) of 12, 5, 1, 0, and 7?
    a. 2
    b. 4
    c. 5
    d. 10

16. $769 + 351 =$
    a. 960
    b. 1,020
    c. 1,080
    d. 1,120

17. If shirts at a garage sale cost $0.75 each, how many shirts can Abby buy for $15.00?
    a. 10
    b. 20
    c. 30
    d. 40

18. If the temperature of the water in a beaker is 60 degrees on the Celsius scale, approximately what is the temperature on the Fahrenheit scale?
    a. 16°F
    b. 32°F
    c. 100°F
    d. 140°F

19. What is the sum of the prime factors of 75?
    a. 5
    b. 8
    c. 13
    d. 18

20. $8,751 - 832 =$
    a. 8,129
    b. 7,919
    c. 9,229
    d. 9,583

21. Which expression is the same as $\dfrac{y^7}{y^4}$?
    a. y^3
    b. $y^{\frac{7}{4}}$
    c. y^{11}
    d. y^{28}

22. $783 \div 27 =$
    a. 29
    b. 33
    c. 37
    d. 39

23. What is 60 percent of 60?
    a. 1
    b. 30
    c. 36
    d. 100

24. If donut holes cost $0.45 for two, how much does it cost to buy 10 donut holes?
    a. $0.90
    b. $1.45
    c. $2.25
    d. $4.50

25. What is the area of a triangle with a base of 10 inches and a height of 9 inches?
    a. 19 sq in
    b. 38 sq in
    c. 45 sq in
    d. 90 sq in

26. If a bowl is 8 inches across at its widest part, what is the area of the circle at the widest part of the bowl?
    a. 8π in^2
    b. 16π in^2
    c. 32π in^2
    d. 64π in^2

27. Express $\dfrac{7}{8}$ as a decimal.
    a. 0.625
    b. 0.875
    c. 62.5
    d. 87.5

28. What are the roots of the equation $x^2 - 7x - 18 = 0$?
    a. $9, -2$
    b. $-4, 9$
    c. $7, 16$
    d. $-2, -4.5$

29. $(4a^2b^4c) \times (-7a^5b^3) =$
    a. $-11a^7b^7c$
    b. $-28a^7b^7c$
    c. $28a^7b^7c$
    d. a^7b^7c

30. What is the sum of the following polynomials?

    $5x + 3xy - 6y^2, 9xy + 7y^2 - 4x$, and $-8y^2 + 7x + 12xy$

    a. $12x + 15xy - 14y^2$
    b. $x + 9xy - 6y^2$
    c. $8x + 24xy - 7y^2$
    d. $5x + 12xy + 7y^2$

31. $3^3 \times 3^2 \times 3^1 =$
    a. 81
    b. 243
    c. 729
    d. 2,187

32. What are the roots of the quadratic equation $3x^2 - x - 10 = 0$?
    a. $x = \sqrt{2}, -5/3$
    b. $x = 2, -\sqrt{5/3}$
    c. $x = -2, \sqrt{5/3}$
    d. $x = 2, -5/3$

33. How many feet to the nearest thousandth would 1 meter contain, if a meter is about 1.094 yards to the nearest thousandth?
    a. 39.75
    b. 3
    c. 3.282
    d. 4.126

34. Express as a polynomial in simple form: $(4x - 2)(2x + 4)$
    a. $6x + 8x - 8$
    b. $6x^2 - 8$
    c. $8x - 20x + 8$
    d. $8x^2 + 12x - 8$

35. Which mathematical property is demonstrated by the following solution?

    $6t - 2 = 22$
    $6t = 24$
    $x = 4$

    a. Distributive property
    b. Inequalities
    c. Factoring polynomials
    d. Equivalent equations

36. The average of two numbers is 20. One number is three-fifths of the other. What are the two numbers?
    a. 15 and 25
    b. 20 and 0
    c. 5 and 8
    d. 30 and 10

37. Express $\dfrac{60}{12}$ as a percentage.

    a. 0.5 percent
    b. 5 percent
    c. 50 percent
    d. 500 percent

38. How many centimeters are in 56 meters?

    a. 56
    b. 560
    c. 5,600
    d. 56,000

39. Jane started her stamp collection exactly one year ago, and in that time, she has collected 132 stamps. On average, how many stamps has she collected per month?

    a. 10
    b. 11
    c. 12
    d. 20

40. $2\dfrac{66}{84} =$

    a. $\dfrac{39}{14}$

    b. $\dfrac{22}{7}$

    c. $\dfrac{85}{21}$

    d. $\dfrac{113}{21}$

Science

45 Minutes

Read each question carefully and then select the correct answer. The correct answers will be found at the end of the test.

1. Phototropism is demonstrated when
   a. a plant grows low to the ground to avoid wind.
   b. light is absorbed by a plant to make energy.
   c. a plant grows toward the sun.
   d. chlorophyll in plant cells causes photosynthesis.

2. An example of a producer in an ecosystem is
   a. a carnivore.
   b. a consumer.
   c. an herbivore.
   d. an algae.

3. A test that creates a photograph of the blood flow in the arteries or veins is called
   a. an angiogram.
   b. an electroencephalogram.
   c. amniocentesis.
   d. an echogram.

4. The boundaries of an ecosystem
   a. constantly change.
   b. are formed by natural barriers.
   c. often overlap other ecosystems.
   d. are limited by the length of its food chains.

5. An ionic bond between two elements involves
   a. shared electrons.
   b. a transfer of electrons.
   c. shared electrons from one element.
   d. a neutral charge.

6. Of the processes below, which one is a different level of defense from the other three?
   a. A low pH in the stomach
   b. Cilia present in the trachea
   c. Cells within the body recognizing a pathogen
   d. Mucus present in the nasal cavity

7. The movement of air through the respiratory system depends on
   a. the movements of the diaphragm.
   b. how hard the muscles in the trachea contract.
   c. how hard the lungs push air out of the body.
   d. cilia along the respiratory tract pushing air in and out of the body.

8. Which pathway/order is correct?
   a. Sperm: testes, epididymis, vas deferens, urethra
   b. Egg: vagina, uterus, ovary, fallopian tube
   c. Development: morula, blastula, zygote, egg
   d. Development: fertilization, ovulation, ejaculation

9. Which of the following statements is false?
   a. Vitamin D and calcium are needed for strong, healthy bones.
   b. Ligaments keep bones joined together.
   c. Skeletal muscle is needed for voluntary movements.
   d. Cartilage's rigidity helps maintain structure.

10. Which of the following statements is false?
    a. The autonomic nervous system allows humans to decide how to use involuntary muscles.
    b. The brain and the spinal cord are part of the central nervous system.
    c. Nerve impulses can send signals faster than chemical signals traveling through the blood.
    d. Neurotransmitters are needed to help send signals between nerves.

11. Inside the kidney one does not find
    a. nephrons.
    b. Bowman's capsules.
    c. glomeruli.
    d. ureters.

12. An amino acid is expected to contain which two functional groups?
    a. $R-NH_2$ and $R-COOH$
    b. $R-CHO$ and $R-CO-NH_2$
    c. $R-OH$ and $R-COOR$
    d. $R-O-R$ and $R-COOH$

13. Which element is most likely to be found in an organic compound?
    a. Carbon
    b. Oxygen
    c. Nitrogen
    d. Calcium

14. Blue litmus paper turns red when the pH of a solution is
    a. 12.
    b. 8.
    c. 6.
    d. 7.

15. When an acid reacts with an active metal such as zinc, the products are
    a. water and salt.
    b. an acid and a base.
    c. neutralized.
    d. a salt and $H_2(g)$.

16. Which of the following substances is most likely to taste sour?
    a. NaOH
    b. NaCl
    c. NH_3
    d. $HC_2H_3O_2$

17. Which of the following reactions demonstrates a neutralization reaction?
    a. $^{232}_{90}Th \rightarrow {}^{228}_{88}Ra + {}^{4}_{2}He$
    b. $NaCl + H_2O \rightarrow HCl + NaOH$
    c. $2HNO_3 + Mg(OH)_2 \rightarrow 2H_2O + Mg(NO_3)_2$
    d. $CH_4 + 2O_2 \rightarrow CO_2 + 2H_2O$

18. The bicuspid valve is found in the
    a. heart.
    b. veins.
    c. lymph nodes.
    d. anus.

19. Which of the following is not an accessory organ?
    a. Liver
    b. Pancreas
    c. Gallbladder
    d. Stomach

20. Bile is stored in the _____ and helps to digest _____ via_____.
    a. liver/proteins/emulsification
    b. liver/fats/dehydration synthesis
    c. gallbladder/fats/emulsification
    d. gallbladder/proteins/proteases

21. If a salt is added to water, which of the following is likely to occur?
    a. The boiling point will increase and the freezing point will decrease.
    b. The boiling point will increase and the freezing point will increase.
    c. The boiling point will decrease and the freezing point will decrease.
    d. The boiling point will decrease and the freezing point will increase.

22. A 60-watt lightbulb is powered by a 110-volt power source. What is the current being drawn?
    a. 1.83 amperes
    b. 0.55 amperes
    c. 50 amperes
    d. 6,600 amperes

23. The kidneys are _____ to the small intestine.
    a. posterior
    b. superior
    c. anterior
    d. medial

24. A protease is an enzyme that works to digest
    a. lipids.
    b. proteins.
    c. carbohydrates.
    d. nucleic acids.

25. Which choice below is in a different category from the other three?
    a. Antibody
    b. Killer T cell
    c. Virus
    d. Phagocytes

26. Breathing occurs through the actions of the
    a. lungs.
    b. nose.
    c. vocal cords.
    d. diaphragm.

27. Which of the following is not a function of the skin?
    a. Providing protection against pathogens
    b. Protecting the body's internal environment
    c. Regulating heat loss
    d. Assisting in the production of white blood cells

28. Which of the following is not a physical part of a nerve cell?
    a. Synapse
    b. Axon
    c. Dendrite
    d. Myelin sheath

29. Metals are malleable and ductile because they have
    a. a lack of electronegativity.
    b. no protons.
    c. ionic crystalline structures.
    d. electron clusters.

30. A solution with a hydrogen ion concentration of 1×10^{-2} M would be classified as
    a. alkali.
    b. neutral.
    c. acid.
    d. base.

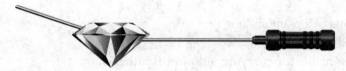

31. The bending of this laser beam of light results from the process called
    a. reflection.
    b. diffraction.
    c. dispersion.
    d. refraction.

32. If the rod cells in an eye were damaged, the nerves of the eye would not be able to transmit
    a. colors.
    b. bright-light conditions.
    c. fine detail.
    d. low-light conditions.

33. The average kinetic energy of a gas remains the same when
    a. its volume is decreased.
    b. its temperature is decreased.
    c. its temperature is increased.
    d. its molecules collide with each other.

34. The human egg is produced in which of these structures of the female reproductive system?
    a. Vagina
    b. Ovary
    c. Uterus
    d. Fallopian tube

35. The purpose of the endocrine system is to
    a. send nerve impulses throughout the body.
    b. aid in digestion.
    c. release chemical signals into the body as to regulate functions.
    d. act as a primary defense against foreign invaders.

36. Plant cells are different from animal cells because plant cells
    a. have a nucleus.
    b. divide to form daughter cells.
    c. have a cell wall.
    d. have no need for chloroplasts.

37. The roots of a plant are not
    a. needed to take up water.
    b. responsible for carrying out photosynthesis.
    c. responsible for anchoring the plant into the soil.
    d. needed to take up minerals from the soil.

38. Which wavelength of light is best absorbed by chlorophyll?
    a. 500 nm
    b. 550 nm
    c. 660 nm
    d. 485 nm

39. Which part of the plant reproductive system is of a different "gender" from the other three?
    a. Stamen
    b. Pistil
    c. Stigma
    d. Style

40. How many times stronger is an acid with a pH of 3 than an acid with a pH of 6?
    a. A pH of 3 is 3 times as strong.
    b. A pH of 3 is 1,000 times as strong.
    c. A pH of 3 is 30 times as weak.
    d. A pH of 3 is 1,000 times as weak.

41. Which of the following is true for a basic solution?
    a. The hydroxide concentration equals zero.
    b. The hydronium concentration equals the hydroxide concentration.
    c. The hydronium concentration is less than the hydroxide concentration.
    d. The hydronium concentration is greater than the hydroxide concentration.

42. A reaction takes place between an acid and 0.5 grams of solid magnesium ribbon. Another reaction takes place between an acid and 0.5 grams of powdered magnesium. Which statement is true?
    a. The powdered magnesium reacts faster because the activation energy has been lowered.
    b. The magnesium strip reacts faster because it has a higher concentration of magnesium.
    c. The powdered magnesium reacts faster because it has a greater surface area.
    d. The magnesium strip reacts faster because it will create a higher temperature once the reaction starts.

43. Two different solutions, A and B, are in separate beakers. These solutions are mixed together in a third beaker that contains pure water. Which statement is true?
    a. The two solutions would have reacted faster if they were mixed together directly and not with water.
    b. The two solutions would react faster if they were under higher pressure.
    c. The two solutions would react faster if they had a greater activation energy.
    d. The two solutions would react faster after being mixed with water because their surface area will be increased.

44. A transverse wave does not have
    a. a compression.
    b. an amplitude.
    c. a frequency.
    d. a wavelength.

45. A wave moves through its medium at 20 m/s with a wavelength of 4 m. What is the frequency of the wave?
    a. 24 s^{-1}
    b. 5 s^{-1}
    c. 16 s^{-1}
    d. 80 s^{-1}

46. Light hits a smooth mirror at an angle of 45°. At what angle will the light be reflected?
    a. 0°
    b. 180°
    c. 45°
    d. 90°

47. White light enters a prism and is broken up into the colors of the rainbow. This phenomenon is called
    a. reflection.
    b. diffraction.
    c. dispersion.
    d. refraction.

48. The alimentary canal is part of the
    a. endocrine system.
    b. nervous system.
    c. digestive system.
    d. reproductive system.

49. A scalar quantity and a vector quantity differ in that
    a. a scalar quantity has both magnitude and direction, and a vector does not.
    b. a scalar quantity has direction only, and a vector has only magnitude.
    c. a vector has both magnitude and direction, and a scalar quantity has only magnitude.
    d. a vector has only direction, and a scalar quantity has only magnitude.

50. Which of the following describes a vector quantity?
    a. Five miles per hour due southwest
    b. Five miles per hour
    c. Five miles
    d. None of the above.

51. An object moves 100 m in 10 s. What is the velocity of the object over this time?
    a. 1,000 m/s
    b. 90 m/s
    c. 110 m/s
    d. 10 m/s

52. An object is moving at 15 m/s. How far will it travel in 5 s?
    a. 75 m
    b. 20 m
    c. 3 m
    d. 15 m

53. An object has a constant velocity of 50 m/s and travels for 10 s. What is the acceleration of the object?
    a. 500 m/s^2
    b. 0 m/s^2
    c. 5 m/s^2
    d. 60 m/s^2

54. The percentage by mass of carbon in CO_2 (formula mass = 44) is
    a. 18 percent.
    b. 27 percent.
    c. 50 percent.
    d. 84 percent.

55. The phloem of a plant transports
    a. food from the roots.
    b. food from the leaves.
    c. water from the roots.
    d. oxygen from cellular respiration.

56. In an experiment designed to determine the rate of photosynthesis in a plant, *Elodea* sprigs were submerged in water in a test tube with sodium bicarbonate. Lightbulbs of different wattages were also used. The distance of the light source was also varied. Changes in volume would indicate the rate of photosynthesis. What would be measured in this experiment to determine photosynthesis?
    a. The amount of CO_2 the plant absorbed from the water
    b. The intensity of the light from different bulbs
    c. The amount of oxygen in the test tube
    d. The temperature changes of the water

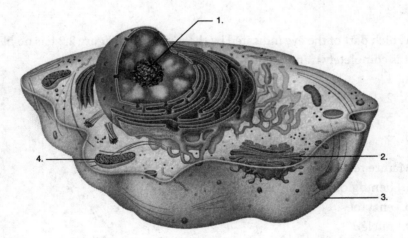

57. Which of the indicated structures in the figure above is the mitochondrion in this animal cell?
    a. 1
    b. 2
    c. 3
    d. 4

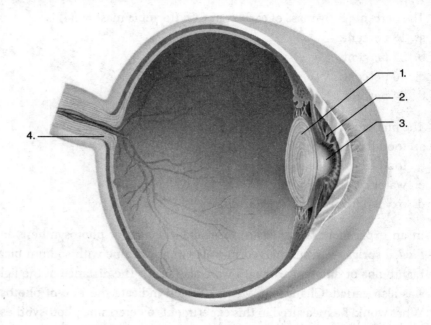

58. The optic nerve is located at what position in the figure above?
    a. 1
    b. 2
    c. 3
    d. 4

59. Which part of the eye indicated by the numbers in Figure 2.3 has no blood cells so it is completely translucent?
    a. 1
    b. 2
    c. 5
    d. 6

60. Mature red blood cells lack
    a. hemoglobin.
    b. enzymes.
    c. nuclei.
    d. leukocytes.

Practice Test 3

Verbal Ability

Word Knowledge and Reading Comprehension

45 minutes

WORD KNOWLEDGE: Read each sentence carefully. Then, on the basis of what is stated in the sentence, select the answer to the incomplete statement. The answers will be found at the end of the test.

1. The young prince felt out of sorts when not in his usual milieu.
   Milieu means
   a. wardrobe.
   b. surroundings.
   c. ancestry.
   d. fortifications.

2. As a neophyte, Terry found camping very difficult.
   Neophyte means
   a. citizen.
   b. surveyor.
   c. connoisseur.
   d. novice.

3. The president of the committee took umbrage at how her work was portrayed in the press. She felt
   a. gratified.
   b. resentful.
   c. discombobulated.
   d. astonished.

4. The lawyer mounted a vociferous defense of her helpless and silent client.
   Vociferous means
   a. defamatory.
   b. convoluted.
   c. strident.
   d. malicious.

5. Everyone felt an air of foreboding when they realized they were lost deep in the woods.
   Foreboding means
   a. humidity.
   b. exuberance.
   c. apprehension.
   d. expectation.

6. Which of the following terms means a torn and ragged wound?
   a. Incision
   b. Abrasion
   c. Lesion
   d. Laceration

7. Which of the following words is a synonym for **blighted**?
   a. Illuminated
   b. Spoiled
   c. Disappointed
   d. Transferred

8. Her first priority as office manager was to _____ the misuse of office supplies.
   a. ignore
   b. curtail
   c. facilitate
   d. replete

9. The costs associated with performing this particular surgery are prohibitive for many hospitals.
   Prohibitive means
   a. excessively high.
   b. dishonest.
   c. forbidden.
   d. understandable.

10. If a patient is surreptitiously eating a bowl of ice cream, he is eating it
    a. stealthily.
    b. quickly.
    c. loudly.
    d. reluctantly.

11. Because of consumer apathy, many gift cards are not cashed in.
    Apathy means
    a. corrosion.
    b. indifference.
    c. avarice.
    d. propriety.

12. In order to keep the location secret, I asked my friends to be
    a. discreet.
    b. disingenuous.
    c. lugubrious.
    d. infantile.

13. For rather seditious reasons, Kevin put the photos up on social networks.
    Seditious means
    a. mundane.
    b. blowsy.
    c. rebellious.
    d. prodigious.

14. The Geiger counter detected some radiation, but the amounts were
    a. ruinous.
    b. negligible.
    c. slanderous.
    d. inexorable.

15. After moving three times in five years, the family was in a state of
    a. animation.
    b. dread.
    c. introspection.
    d. flux.

16. Her mother-in-law offered several gibes, which she chose to ignore.
    Gibes means
    a. confessions.
    b. insults.
    c. exaggerations.
    d. aphorisms.

READING COMPREHENSION: There are five reading passages in this section. Read each passage carefully. Then, on the basis of what you have read in the passage, select the best answer for each question.

PASSAGE 1

A land bridge is land exposed when the sea recedes, connecting one expanse of land to another. One of the most famous land bridges was the Bering Land Bridge, often known as Beringia, which connected Alaska to Siberia across what is now the Bering Strait.

The Bering Land Bridge was not terribly long. If it still existed today, you could drive across it in your car in about an hour. It appeared during the Ice Age, when enormous sheets of ice covered much of Europe and America. The ice sheets contained huge amounts of water north of the Equator, and because of this, the sea level dropped precipitously, perhaps as much as 400 feet, revealing landmasses such as the Bering Land Bridge.

At this time, the ecology of the Northern Hemisphere was that of the Mammoth Steppe. It was a dry, frigid land filled with grasses, sedges, and tundra vegetation. It supported many large grazing animals, including reindeer, bison, and musk oxen, as well as the lions that fed upon them. It also contained large camels, giant short-faced bears, and woolly mammoths. Many of the animals of the Mammoth Steppe used the bridge to cross from east to west and back again. Eventually, their human hunters tracked them from Asia to North America.

Ethnologists and geologists generally believe that humans used the Bering Land Bridge to populate the Americas, which up until about 24,000 years ago had no sign of human life. Ethnologists use such evidence as shared religions, similar houses and tools, and unique methods of cleaning and preserving food to show the link between the people of coastal Siberia and the people of coastal Alaska.

There are those among the Native American population who dispute the land bridge theory. For one thing, it contradicts most native teachings on the origins of the people. For another, it seems to undermine the notion that they are truly "native" to the North American continent.

17. According to this passage, the first people in North America lived
    a. in what is now Central America.
    b. west of the Bering Strait.
    c. below sea level.
    d. in what is now Alaska.

18. Based on information in the passage, about how long was the Bering Land Bridge?
    a. Between 50 and 75 miles long
    b. Between 90 and 120 miles long
    c. Around 150 miles long
    d. Around 200 miles long

19. According to the passage, which of these would be considered a land bridge?
    a. The Isthmus of Panama
    b. The Chesapeake Bay
    c. The Strait of Hormuz
    d. The Khyber Pass

20. In the third paragraph, the author includes information about large mammals in order to
    a. explain patterns of growth among animals of the Mammoth Steppe.
    b. indicate how tough animals needed to be to survive the Ice Age.
    c. contrast the climate of North America with the climate of Asia.
    d. suggest a reason for human migration from Asia to North America.

21. The author's purpose in the fourth paragraph is to
    a. introduce a theory and show some support for it.
    b. compare some processes used by geologists and ethnologists.
    c. list some possible reasons for the migrations of early humans.
    d. contradict a theory about an early use of the land bridge.

22. The author suggests that some contemporary Native Americans object to the land bridge theory because
    a. it equates them with Pleistocene man.
    b. it challenges their history and status.
    c. it relies on disputed science.
    d. it downplays the importance of southern tribes.

PASSAGE 2

One of the most common stereotypes surrounding young teenage boys is that they are hostile, belligerent, and generally display "attitude." Some considered this just a phase in the maturing process, some thought it was a reflection of poor parenting skills, and others placed blame on everything from violent video games to too much television.

A recent study by a team of Australian and American researchers may prove all of those theories wrong. These researchers say that boys' aggressive behaviors may actually be due to overly large amygdalae in the boys' brains. The amygdala is a part of the brain found deep within the medial temporal lobes. It is intricately involved in emotional responses such as fear and anger.

As the researchers reported in an article for the *Proceedings of the National Academy of Science,* boys may show no ability to control their emotions because they literally do not have the brain development to do so until their early twenties. According to Nicholas Allen of the University of Melbourne's psychology department, "It's important to realize that . . . parts of the brain are still developing for these young people."

The study required 137 twelve-year-old boys and their parents to sit down and discuss emotionally sensitive issues, such as homework, bedtime, and hours spent on the Internet. Afterwards, the boys' brains were scanned. Boys who had the largest amygdalae behaved more aggressively than other boys who had smaller ones. They also appeared to have smaller-than-usual prefrontal cortexes, the region of the brain that is involved with regulating emotions.

The researchers concluded that those boys who had less brain development had a much stronger tendency to be negative and even hostile when they interacted with their parents. Just do not tell the teenage boys—it gives them a built-in excuse!

23. Which of these topics is the main focus of the passage?
    a. How best to discipline unruly young people
    b. Why scientists think that the amygdala affects emotions
    c. How behavior may be linked to brain development
    d. Why parents and teenage boys tend to have disagreements

24. According to the study, when is brain development sufficient for boys to control their emotions?
    a. By the time boys reach puberty
    b. By the time boys reach their mid-to-late teens
    c. By the time boys graduate from high school
    d. By the time boys reach their early twenties

25. Why does the author include a quote from Nicholas Allen?
    a. His son is one of the boys involved in the study.
    b. His credentials lend authority to the conclusions of the study.
    c. He himself was once an overly aggressive young man.
    d. He was the one who initiated the research study.

26. What physical tests were performed after the boys and their parents discussed sensitive issues?
    a. The boys' brains were scanned.
    b. The boys' blood was analyzed for elevated testosterone levels.
    c. The parents' blood pressure levels were measured.
    d. The boys were given MRIs.

27. What conclusion did researchers reach about boys with "attitude"?
    a. The boys would benefit from additional discipline from parents.
    b. Surgery and medication would be beneficial in controlling emotions.
    c. Brain development was the key to much of their overall behavior.
    d. Additional research is needed to find out how to prevent brain abnormalities.

28. Which summary best matches the author's main point?
    a. Smaller amygdalae lead to more aggressive behavior.
    b. More brain development causes a much stronger tendency to be negative and even hostile.
    c. Shrinking amygdalae lead to less aggressive behavior.
    d. Less brain development causes a much stronger tendency to be negative and even hostile.

PASSAGE 3

Lie out in the sun too much today and get skin cancer 20 years from now. Smoke too many cigarettes now and get lung cancer decades down the road. Now there is potentially a third danger to add to this list: be exposed to too much lead, pesticides, or mercury now and have your aging brain become seriously confused during your senior years.

"We're trying to offer a caution that a portion of what has been called normal aging might in fact be due to ubiquitous environmental exposures like lead," says Dr. Brian Schwartz of Johns Hopkins University. "The fact that it's happening with lead is the first proof of the principle that it's possible."

A new area of medical research is one that studies how exposure to toxic elements in younger years can result in serious health problems in senior years. It is difficult to research these problems because the only way to do so is to observe people over many years to determine results.

Physicians test for lead amounts by seeing how much has accumulated in a person's shinbone. Testing the blood also often reveals amounts of lead, but that is a sign of recent, not lifelong, exposure. The higher the lifetime lead dose, according to the study, the worse the performance of mental functions, including verbal and visual memory and language ability.

29. What is the best title for this passage?
    a. There Is Lead Everywhere
    b. The Shins Tell a Story
    c. Toxins Today, Health Problems Tomorrow
    d. Avoid the Sun—and Cigarette Smoke

30. You might infer from this passage that
    a. people may be exposed to lead more than they realize.
    b. doctors are increasingly concerned about what happens to the brain during aging.
    c. shinbones are good indicators of many health ailments or conditions.
    d. blood tests are the best way to measure individuals' lifetime lead exposure.

31. Why is the effect of lead exposure hard to study?
    a. Lead is difficult to trace in the body.
    b. Today, exposure to lead is no longer a problem.
    c. Lead is discarded from the body at too rapid a rate.
    d. Scientists have to observe lead exposure in subjects over a long time period.

32. Why does the author of the article include a quote from Dr. Brian Schwartz?
    a. To point out how exposure to several toxins can affect the brain
    b. To support the idea that some symptoms of aging might be due to lead exposure
    c. To introduce an idea that contradicts the main point of the article
    d. To demonstrate that all doctors are taking this new research on lead seriously

33. What conclusion can be drawn from the fact that the shinbone is used for diagnosing lead levels?
    a. Lead accumulates only in the shinbone.
    b. The shin bone is very delicate.
    c. Lead stays within the body for a long time.
    d. It is easiest to test bones that are not in constant use.

34. Why don't scientists just do a long-term study to determine the effects of lead exposure on humans?
    a. It would take years to be sure whether they should warn people.
    b. Lead does not remain in the body for that long a time.
    c. It is not possible to test people over a long period of time.
    d. Lead is found in the blood, and blood changes over time.

PASSAGE 4

Everyone knows that pepper is great for adding a little extra flavor to food, but a new study from Great Britain says that it may also have a medicinal purpose. Apparently, black pepper can help treat a disfiguring skin condition known as vitiligo.

Vitiligo is a disease that kills the skin's melanin, the element that gives skin its color and protects it from the sun's ultraviolet (UV) rays. It is the condition that the late pop star Michael Jackson said was responsible for changes in his skin color.

Researchers at King's College in London studied piperine, the compound in pepper that gives the spice its unique spicy flavor. Apparently piperine, along with its synthetic derivatives, helps stimulate pigmentation in people's skin, especially when phototherapy treatment is combined with UV radiation.

To date, treatment for vitiligo has consisted of steroids applied directly to the skin as well as phototherapy. However, a number of people do not respond effectively to hormones, and phototherapy always carries with it a risk of skin cancer. Piperine, on the other hand, when applied to the skin resulted in an even brown color within a mere six weeks.

35.   The best title for this selection is
       a. Pepper Always Adds Flavor.
       b. No Cure Yet for Vitiligo.
       c. Pepper Provides Pigmentation.
       d. Pepper's Piperine.

36.   What substance were the scientists studying?
       a. Piperine
       b. Melanin
       c. Pigmentation
       d. Phototherapy

37.   Piperine gives pepper its
       a. color.
       b. flavor.
       c. aroma.
       d. shape.

38.   What is one of the main functions of melanin?
       a. To keep the skin supple
       b. To release hormones
       c. To provide taste
       d. To protect from UV rays

39.   Which treatment seems to have the highest risk?
       a. Piperine
       b. Phototherapy
       c. Steroids
       d. Hormones

40. It can be inferred from the passage that
    a. Michael Jackson suffered from a piperine deficiency.
    b. hormone treatment can cause cancer in some people.
    c. steroids are one form of phototherapy that is effective.
    d. doctors are not applying ground pepper to people's skin.

PASSAGE 5

The Arecibo Observatory, near the north shore of Puerto Rico, is a key component of Cornell University's National Astronomy and Ionosphere Center (NAIC). In a joint venture with the National Science Foundation, the observatory exists to provide observation time and support for scientists worldwide. A panel of judges determines the "most promising" research proposals among the hundreds that are presented to the observatory each year. Those scientists are invited to Puerto Rico for viewing time on Arecibo's giant telescope.

Scientists who visit the observatory are typically involved in one of three studies: radio astronomy, which is the study of natural radio energy produced by faraway galaxies and stars; atmospheric science, which is the study of the Earth's upper atmosphere, including its temperature, density, and composition; and radar astronomy, which is the study of planets and their moons, asteroids, and comets. The enormous telescope assists with all three studies.

The Arecibo telescope does not resemble what most of us think of when we hear the word *telescope*. Its reflective surface covers a remarkable 20 acres. Dangling above it are towers and cables, subreflectors and antennas, all of which can be positioned using 26 motors to transmit radio waves and receive echoes with astonishing precision.

Arecibo has been the site of hundreds of fascinating discoveries. Among these are the rate of rotation of the planet Mercury, determined two years after the telescope launched in 1963; two new classes of pulsars; and the first planets ever spotted outside of our solar system. Today, one of the most important goals of the observatory is to document and quantify global climate change by monitoring changes in temperature, hydrogen composition, and wind-fields in the ionosphere.

Although at one time scientists had to travel to Puerto Rico to share viewing time on the giant telescope, today there are new protocols that enable remote viewing. At the University of Texas at Brownsville, students are helping to design a remote-control command center that will control the positioning of the telescope from 2,000 miles away. Students and professors will use the command center to study radio pulsars, rotating neutron stars that release radiation in regular pulses.

41. In the context of the second paragraph, the word **composition** means
    a. structure.
    b. array.
    c. opus.
    d. compilation.

42. Based on the information in the third paragraph, you can conclude that most telescopes
    a. do not have reflective surfaces.
    b. contain radio antennas.
    c. are not as large as Arecibo's.
    d. cannot be repositioned.

43. All of these are typical studies at Arecibo *except*
    a. the nature of the ionosphere.
    b. the production of remote-control devices.
    c. radio waves produced by galaxies.
    d. investigations of distant asteroids.

44. The author's purpose in the fourth paragraph is to
    a. provide the history of the observatory.
    b. describe Arecibo in some detail.
    c. compare and contrast astronomical studies.
    d. list some of Arecibo's successes.

45. Which statement expresses a personal opinion?
    a. "Those scientists are invited to Puerto Rico for viewing time on Arecibo's giant telescope."
    b. "Scientists who visit the observatory are typically involved in one of three studies."
    c. "Arecibo has been the site of hundreds of fascinating discoveries."
    d. "Students and professors will use the command center to study radio pulsars."

46. The remote-control command center will *most* likely
    a. result in fewer significant research findings.
    b. save scientists the cost of traveling.
    c. fail to achieve its goal of assisting students.
    d. be used primarily for atmospheric studies.

WORD KNOWLEDGE: Read each sentence carefully. Then, on the basis of what is stated in the sentence, select the answer to the incomplete statement. The answers will be found at the end of the test.

47. Specific criteria for these grants kept them from being awarded for capricious reasons.
    Capricious means
    a. flawless.
    b. malicious.
    c. impulsive.
    d. reconsidered.

48. A dog can often prevent poisoning by being able to regurgitate food it has eaten.

    Regurgitate means to
    a. digest.
    b. vomit.
    c. neutralize.
    d. convert.

49. After 62 days wandering in the desert, Brenda emerged looking
    a. cadaverous.
    b. nostalgic.
    c. resilient.
    d. palliative.

50. The new office building had so many walls and hallways that it felt like a(n)
    a. auditorium.
    b. labyrinth.
    c. podium.
    d. paroxysm.

51. The difference between two elements or issues is often referred to as a(n)
    a. efficacy.
    b. disparity.
    c. impunity.
    d. unction.

52. As she read the letter, the frown on her face was gradually supplanted by a smile.

    Supplanted means
    a. replaced.
    b. vindicated.
    c. coerced.
    d. supported.

53. The handsome new intern had an entourage behind him every step of the way.

    Entourage means
    a. students.
    b. followers.
    c. rivals.
    d. nurses.

54. If history has taught us nothing else, it is that humans are consistently fallible.

    Fallible means
    a. gullible.
    b. amusing.
    c. imperfect.
    d. immortal.

55. If the hospital staff considers the head surgeon to be a venerable doctor, it means they considered her to be
    a. well respected.
    b. pleasant in nature.
    c. attractive in appearance.
    d. intimidating.

56. The new administrative assistant had a talent for quickly and accurately assessing situations and people; she was thought to be quite
    a. astute.
    b. diffident.
    c. courageous.
    d. corpulent.

57. Which of the following words is a synonym for **deride**?
    a. Ignore
    b. Influence
    c. Ridicule
    d. Bolster

58. The speaker had a habit of losing focus; he would routinely _____ to unrelated topics.
    a. digress
    b. regress
    d. condescend
    d. elaborate

59. Which of the following words means the opposite of **supple**?
    a. Rigid
    b. Pliant
    c. Elongated
    d. Curly

60. Nurse Dickson, who had lost all enthusiasm for her work, spoke to all the new volunteers in a very prosaic manner.
    Prosaic means
    a. inspirational.
    b. complicated.
    c. commonplace.
    d. imaginative.

Mathematics

45 Minutes

Work each problem carefully. Use scrap paper to do your calculations. The correct answers will be found at the end of the test.

1. $14,985 + 3,806 =$
   a. 17,781
   b. 17,791
   c. 18,781
   d. 18,791

Use this chart to answer questions 2 and 3.

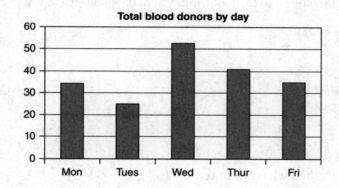

2. What is the approximate percent increase between the number of donors on Tuesday and the number of donors on Wednesday?
   a. 255 percent
   b. 50 percent
   c. 100 percent
   d. 200 percent

3. Which day showed the largest decrease in the number of blood donors from the day before?
   a. Tuesday
   b. Wednesday
   c. Thursday
   d. Friday

4. $5,263 - 3,959 =$
   a. 1,304
   b. 1,394
   c. 1,404
   d. 1,494

5. What is the average (arithmetic mean) of 23, 8, 2, and 7?
   a. 4.5
   b. 7.5
   c. 8
   d. 10

6. Express $\dfrac{7}{35}$ as a decimal.
   a. 0.014
   b. 0.14
   c. 0.02
   d. 0.2

7. What is the solution to the following system of equations? $x + y = 4$ and $2x - 6y = 3$
   a. $x = -\dfrac{27}{8}, y = \dfrac{5}{8}$
   b. $x = \dfrac{27}{8}, y = -\dfrac{5}{8}$
   c. $x = \dfrac{27}{8}, y = \dfrac{5}{8}$
   d. $x = -\dfrac{27}{8}, y = \dfrac{8}{5}$

8. If $\sqrt[3]{x} = y^4$, then what is x in terms of y?
   a. $x = y^{12}$
   b. $x = y^7$
   c. $x = y^4$
   d. $x = y$

9. A bag of candies contains 10 red, 9 yellow, 8 orange, 6 green, and 4 blue colored candies. What is the probability of randomly choosing an orange-colored candy from the bag?
   a. $\dfrac{8}{37}$
   b. $\dfrac{37}{8}$
   c. $\dfrac{8}{27}$
   d. $\dfrac{3}{4}$

10. What is the probability of selecting an ace of a red suit from a standard deck of cards?

    a. $\dfrac{1}{52}$

    b. $\dfrac{2}{52}$

    c. $\dfrac{48}{52}$

    d. $\dfrac{50}{52}$

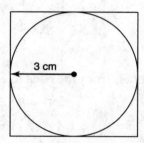

3 cm

11. What is the area of the square in the diagram?
    a. 12 cm²
    b. 36 cm²
    c. 6 cm²
    d. 24 cm²

12. Doris is leaning a 10-foot ladder against a wall. If the ladder hits the wall at exactly 8 feet, how far away from the wall is the ladder placed on the floor?
    a. 2 ft
    b. 6 ft
    c. 8 ft
    d. 10 ft

13. What is the average (arithmetic mean) of 8, 3, 6, and 11?
    a. 4
    b. 6
    c. 7
    d. 9

14. If Melanie can complete 6 forms in 15 minutes, how long will it take her to complete 30 forms?
    a. 12 min.
    b. 60 min.
    c. 75 min.
    d. 120 min.

15. $3,892 + 364 =$
    a. 4,126
    b. 4,156
    c. 4,256
    d. 5,254

16. If Ryan is two years older than four times the age of his dog, Pixie, which expression represents that relationship?
    a. $R = 4 + 2P$
    b. $R = (2 + 4)P$
    c. $R = R = \dfrac{2+4}{P}$
    d. $R = 2 + 4P$

17. If the longest distance across from the edge to edge of a circle is 10 feet, what is the area of the circle?
    a. 5 ft
    b. 25π ft^2
    c. 50π ft^2
    d. 100π ft^2

18. The measurement from the center to the rim of an economy car tire is 15 inches. How much road can this tire cover in one rotation?
    a. 30π in
    b. 180π in
    c. 225π in
    d. 360π in

19. Linda is making a smoothie recipe that calls for five parts berries to four parts yogurt. If she puts in 10 cups of yogurt for a big party, how many cups of berries will she need?
    a. 2.5
    b. 5
    c. 10
    d. 12.5

20. If the number of babies born in a certain maternity ward in January is five more than twice the number born in February, which of the following mathematical statements reflects this relationship?
    a. $J = 2 + 5F$
    b. $J = (5 + 2)F$
    c. $J = 5 + 2F$
    d. $J = (2 + 5)F$

21. If the annual operating expenses of a corporation are graphed in a pie chart and building maintenance accounts for $33\frac{1}{3}$ percent, what is the measure of the central angle that represents this percentage?
    a. 80°
    b. 10°
    c. 120°
    d. 180°

22. Fred is trying to determine the longest line that can be drawn on a presentation board, and he has determined that it must be the diagonal of the board. If the board is 4 feet by 6 feet, what is the length of its diagonal?
    a. $\sqrt{15}$
    b. $16\sqrt{3}$
    c. $2\sqrt{13}$
    d. $4\sqrt{5}$

23. Completely simplify $\sqrt{80}$.
    a. $2\sqrt{5}$
    b. $4\sqrt{5}$
    c. $2\sqrt{20}$
    d. $4\sqrt{20}$

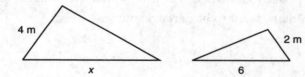

24. How many meters is x? Assume the triangles are similar with corresponding sides.
    a. 12 m
    b. 15 m
    c. 24 m
    d. 5 m

25. Michelle can paint two walls in 90 minutes. How long will it take her paint six walls?
    a. 30 min.
    b. 45 min.
    d. 180 min.
    d. 270 min.

26. $5.31 \div 3 =$
    a. 1.77
    b. 1.79
    c. 1.97
    d. 1.99

27. 329 × 43 =
   a. 11,347
   b. 12,947
   c. 14,147
   d. 15,237

28. If Andy receives 20 percent of the retail price on each of his published books, how much does he make on a book that retails for $35?
   a. $5
   b. $7
   c. $14
   d. $28

29. Express $\dfrac{60}{24}$ as a percentage.
   a. 25 percent
   b. 40 percent
   c. 250 percent
   d. 400 percent

30. After surveying her fellow nursing school students, Amber has found that the ratio of students who want to be surgical nurses compared with those who want to be geriatric nurses is 5:2. If 30 of her classmates want to be surgical nurses, how many want to be geriatric nurses?
   a. 10
   b. 12
   c. 15
   d. 18

31. 583 × 6 =
   a. 3,480
   b. 1,758
   c. 3,378
   d. 3,498

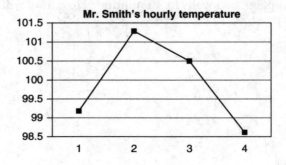

32. In which hour did Mr. Smith's temperature change the most?
    a. 1-2
    b. 2-3
    c. 3-4
    d. 4-5

33. Dora is three years younger than half the age of one of her regular patients, Mario. Which of the following mathematical statements reflects this relationship?
    a. $D = 2M + 3$
    b. $D = 2M - 3$
    c. $D = \frac{1}{2}M + 3$
    d. $D = \frac{1}{2}M - 3$

34. The number 5 is what percent of 40?
    a. 8
    b. 12.5
    c. 80
    d. 125

35. $7,314 \div 46 =$
    a. 159
    b. 159 r4
    c. 262
    d. 262 r6

36. Upon rolling a pair of dice, what is the probability that the sum of the two numbers on the dice is either 7 or 12?
    a. $\dfrac{1}{6}$
    b. $\dfrac{1}{36}$
    c. $\dfrac{5}{36}$
    d. $\dfrac{7}{36}$

37. What is the probability that two cards drawn from a deck of cards are of a black suit (e.g., either clubs or spades) if the first card drawn is replaced before the second card is drawn?
    a. $\dfrac{1,352}{2,704}$
    b. $\dfrac{676}{2,704}$
    c. $\dfrac{6}{2,704}$
    d. $\dfrac{2}{2,704}$

38. Chemistry students performed nine volume measurements of a solution during a lab and obtained the following results: {2.4 mL, 3.2 mL, 3.7 mL, 3.7 mL, 4.5 mL, 6.8 mL, 7.3 mL, 8.1 mL, 12.2 mL}. What is the mean of the data set to the nearest tenth milliliter?

a. 3.7 mL
b. 4.5 mL
c. 5.8 mL
d. 9.8 mL

39. What is the median of the data set?

a. 3.7 mL
b. 4.5 mL
c. 5.8 mL
d. 9.8 mL

40. What is the mode of the data set?

a. 3.7 mL
b. 4.5 mL
c. 5.8 mL
d. 9.8 mL

Science

45 Minutes

Read each question carefully and then select the correct answer. The correct answers will be found at the end of the test.

1. When calculating an object's acceleration, you must
    a. divide the change in time by the velocity.
    b. multiply the velocity and time.
    c. find the difference between the time and velocity.
    d. divide the change in velocity by the change in time.

2. Which of these objects has the least amount of momentum?
    a. A 1,250-kg car moving at 5 m/s
    b. A 0.5-kg rock rolling at 40 m/s
    c. A 10-kg piece of meteorite moving at 600 m/s
    d. An 80-kg person running at 4 m/s

3. Momentum is calculated using the formula
    a. $F = ma$
    b. $p = mv$
    c. $\dfrac{1}{2} mv^2$
    d. $q = H_v m$

4. The unit of measure of momentum is
    a. m/s.
    b. m/s^2.
    c. kg·m/s.
    d. N·m/s.

5. Newtons (N) are measured in
    a. m/s.
    b. watts.
    c. kg.
    d. kg·m/s^2.

6. The six different cells of the stomach lining produce different substances to aid digestion. Which of these produced would digest proteins?
    a. Pepsin enzymes
    b. Gastic mucus
    c. Gastrin hormones
    d. Hydrogen and chloride ions

7. The vessel carrying blood from the heart to the body is called the
   a. vena cava.
   b. pulmonary artery.
   c. aorta.
   d. left ventricle.

8. A photon is a
   a. valence-level electron.
   b. neutrino.
   c. light particle.
   d. quark.

9. The resistance in an alternating current series circuit is 9 ohms. If the potential difference across this circuit is 27.0 volts, what would the current be?
   a. 0.243 amperes
   b. 36 amperes
   c. 18 amperes
   d. 3 amperes

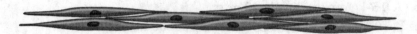

10. Where in the body would smooth muscles tissues of this type be found?
    a. The heart
    b. The intestine
    c. The gluteus maximus
    d. The tongue

11. The major difference between smooth muscles and other types is
    a. a lack of striations.
    b. only one nucleus in each cell.
    c. nuclei in each fiber.
    d. the presence of striations.

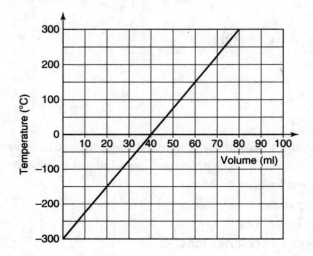

12. The volume and temperature of an ideal gas are shown plotted against each other in this graph. When the volume of the gas increases from 40 ml to 70 ml, the temperature changes by about
    a. 30°C.
    b. 50°C.
    c. 142°C.
    d. 220°C.

13. Through which medium would sound move the fastest?
    a. A glass rod
    b. An iron pipe
    c. A swimming pool's water
    d. A wooden floor

14. What is the fourth state of matter?
    a. Crystal
    b. Ionic
    c. Plasma
    d. Zeolite

15. A glass brick is
    a. transparent.
    b. translucent.
    c. reflective.
    d. opaque.

16. Which of the following methods of medical imaging uses magnetism?
    a. Radiography
    b. CT
    c. Ultrasound
    d. MRI

17. The bones of the human body have many functions except
    a. protecting organs.
    b. creating blood cells.
    c. providing movement.
    d. storing minerals.

18. A car travels 3 miles north, 6 miles south, 2 miles east, 2 miles west, and then 3 miles north. Which of the following is *true*?
    a. The displacement of the car is 16 miles, and the distance traveled is 0 miles.
    b. The displacement of the car is 16 miles, and the distance traveled is 16 miles.
    c. The displacement of the car is 0 miles, and the distance traveled is 0 miles.
    d. The displacement of the car is 0 miles, and the distance traveled is 16 miles.

19. A car is traveling at 5 miles per second. A squirrel jumps into the middle of the road, and the car comes to a screeching halt over 2.5 seconds. What is the car's acceleration over this time period?
    a. -2 m/s^2
    b. 2 m/s^2
    c. 1.25 m/s^2
    d. 0 m/s^2

20. A car, starting from rest, accelerates at 10 meters for 5 seconds. What is the velocity of the car after 5 seconds?
    a. 2 m/s
    b. 50 m/s
    c. 0 m/s
    d. The answer cannot be determined from the information given.

21. Which of these objects has the greatest momentum?
    a. A 1,250-kg car moving at 5 m/s
    b. A 0.5-kg rock moving at 40 m/s
    c. A 10-kg piece of meteorite moving at 600 m/s
    d. An 80-kg person running at 4 m/s

22. A 1.0-kg block on a table is given a push so that it slides along the table. If the block is accelerated at 6 m/s^2, then what was the force applied to the block?
    a. 3 N
    b. 0 N
    c. 6 N
    d. The answer cannot be determined from the information given.

23. A box is moved by a 15-N force over a distance of 3 meters. What is the amount of work that has been done?
    a. 450 C
    b. 5 J
    c. 45 W
    d. 45 N·m

24. Which of the following is true?
    a. The amplitude of a wave is the distance that one complete wave covers.
    b. The frequency of a wave is the distance the crests and troughs are from the normal.
    c. The wavelength of a wave is how many waves pass a point in a given amount of time.
    d. The velocity of a wave can be found by multiplying the frequency by the wavelength.

25. Which of the following is *not* correctly paired up with its unit of measure?
    a. Current/Ohms
    b. Voltage/Volts
    c. Charge/Coulombs
    d. Power/Watts

26. The symbol Ω represents
    a. current.
    b. resistance.
    c. amperes.
    d. power.

27. Which equation is written incorrectly, demonstrating a relationship that does not exist?
    a. $V = IR$
    b. $P = IV$
    c. $R = V/I$
    d. $I = R/V$

28. A set of lights decorates the window of a store. One of the lightbulbs burns out, but the remaining lightbulbs stay lit. The lightbulbs are connected in
    a. parallel.
    b. series.
    c. short circuit.
    d. a 220-volt line.

29. What is the voltage required to deliver a current of 1.0 amps to a device that has a resistance of 1.5 ohms?
    a. 2.5 V
    b. 1.5 V
    c. 0.67 V
    d. 0.5 V

30. Electrical potential is measured in
    a. ohms.
    b. watts.
    c. amperes.
    d. volts.

31. Newton's first law describes
    a. inertia.
    b. acceleration.
    c. forces.
    d. apples.

32. Newton's second law describes
    a. inertia.
    b. acceleration.
    c. quantum mechanics.
    d. relativity.

33. Newton's third law describes
    a. inertia.
    b. static friction.
    c. forces.
    d. string theory.

34. An object sliding along a table top will come to rest because of
    a. a gain in potential energy.
    b. a gain in kinetic energy.
    c. a force of friction.
    d. an increase in momentum.

35. A force of 3 N is applied to a box, causing it to move 5 meters. What is the amount of work done?
    a. 15 N·kg
    b. 15 N/m
    c. 15 N·m
    d. 15 N·m/s^2

36. One hundred N·m of work is done over 20 meters. What force was applied to the object that was moved?
    a. 120 N
    b. 5 N
    c. 80 N
    d. 2,000 N

37. A book is held 6 feet above the floor and then dropped. Which statement is *true*?
    a. The potential energy of the book is converted to kinetic energy.
    b. The potential energy of the book is destroyed.
    c. Kinetic energy is created.
    d. The total energy of the system will not be conserved.

38. The joule cannot be the unit for
    a. potential energy.
    b. kinetic energy.
    c. heat energy.
    d. height.

39. Which organ below has olfactory cells?
    a. Nose
    b. Ear
    c. Tongue
    d. Eye

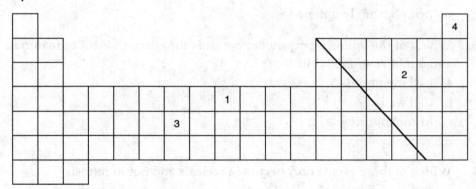

40. On the periodic table shown above, the noble gases are located around
    a. 1.
    b. 2.
    c. 3.
    d. 4.

41. Which of the various mediums of different refractive indices shown below would offer yellow light the least resistance?
    a. 1.00
    b. 1.47
    c. 1.33
    d. 2.42

42. In order to gather material for genetic testing, scientists cannot gather material from human beings. They can, however,
    a. draw family trees that trace certain diseases among related individuals.
    b. view human eggs with a microscope.
    c. detail genetic characteristics from individuals.
    d. place human eggs in a petri dish and fertilize them.

43. Which of the following statements is true?
    a. DNA is made of amino acids.
    b. RNA is double-stranded.
    c. Cytosine replaces uracil in RNA.
    d. Thymine pairs with adenine in DNA.

44. The genotype and phenotype for human life are determined by which of the following organic compounds?
    a. Water
    b. Carbohydrates
    c. Nucleic acids
    d. Amino acids

45. Which of the following transports oxygen in human blood?
    a. Phagocytes and white blood cells
    b. Hemoglobin in red blood cells
    c. Platelets
    d. Lymph from lymph nodes

46. Which of the following organelles controls the entry and exit of materials into and out of an animal cell?
    a. Cell membrane
    b. Cell wall
    c. Mitochondrion
    d. Vacuole

47. Which of these events only occurs in meiosis and not in mitosis?
    a. Following replication, each chromosome is made of two chromatids.
    b. Homologous chromosomes move to the spindle individually.
    c. Identical sets of chromosomes move in opposite directions.
    d. After cell division, each cell has only two chromosomes.

48. The parts of the eye that allow humans to see colors and make out objects in low light conditions are the
    a. rods and cones.
    b. lens.
    c. corneas.
    d. optic nerves.

49. When a diver leaps from a cliff and plunges into the water below, what levels of energy are reached as she hits the water?
    a. The greatest potential energy
    b. Buildup of gravitational potential energy with some kinetic energy
    c. Maximum kinetic energy and no gravitational potential energy
    d. No kinetic energy or gravitational potential energy

50. When electrical charges are rearranged on an object without touching it, this is called
    a. friction.
    b. conduction.
    c. insulation.
    d. induction.

51. Patients with diabetes are likely to have
    a. a high level of glucose in their urine.
    b. almost no glucose in their urine.
    c. a low blood-sugar level.
    d. normal blood-sugar levels.

52. The sky is blue during the day and not at sunset because
    a. there is no dust in the air during the day to block colors.
    b. the sun's heat is more intense and clears the air.
    c. sunlight is travelling through more air and other colors are blocked.
    d. sunlight is travelling through less air at noon than at sunset.

53. When white light is broken into the colors of the rainbow, _____ occurs.
    a. reflection
    b. dispersion
    c. refraction
    d. diffraction

54. Referring to Ohm's law, you can conclude that
    a. voltage and current are inversely proportional when resistance is constant.
    b. an electronic device that is connected to a 6-volt source and draws 3 amperes has a total resistance of 2 ohms.
    c. resistance is measured in volts.
    d. voltage is the amount of charge that passes through a point per second.

55. Newton's second law is shown by which of the following equations?
    a. $PV = nRT$
    b. $F = ma$
    c. $p = mv$
    d. $a = v/t$

56. The bending of light that takes place as light passes from air to quartz is called
    a. deflection.
    b. diffraction.
    c. refraction.
    d. absorption.

57. A 110-volt appliance draws 2.0 amperes. How many watts of power does it require?
    a. 220 W
    b. 55 W
    c. 112 W
    d. 108 W

58. A 110-volt hair dryer delivers 1,525 watts of power. How many amperes does it draw?
    a. 167,750 A
    b. 1,635 A
    c. 1,415 A
    d. 13.9 A

59. A force of 10 N is delivered to an object for 1.5 seconds. What is the impulse directed on the object?
    a. 15 N·s
    b. 8.5 N
    c. 11.5 s
    d. 6.7 N/s

60. A 10-kilogram object moving at 5 meters per second has an impulse acted on it, causing the velocity to change to 15 meters per second. What was the impulse applied to the object?
    a. 10 kg·m/s
    b. 20 kg·m/s
    c. 15 kg·m/s
    d. 100 kg·m/s

Practice Test 4

Verbal Ability
Word Knowledge and Reading Comprehension

45 Minutes

WORD KNOWLEDGE: Read each sentence carefully. Then, on the basis of what is stated in the sentence, select the answer to the incomplete statement. The answers will be found at the end of the test.

1. On that rainy afternoon, lying on that comfortable couch, she was filled with a pervasive feeling of
   a. ambition.
   b. indolence.
   c. turmoil.
   d. frustration.

2. The sorrowful look on her face was a harbinger of bad news.
   Harbinger means
   a. bigot.
   b. servant.
   c. messenger.
   d. charlatan.

3. The woman spent 10 minutes extolling the virtues of her favorite plastic surgeon.
   Extolling means
   a. commending.
   b. fixating on.
   c. censoring.
   d. denying.

4. The crew worked for hours endeavoring to extricate the passengers trapped in the stalled elevator.
   Endeavoring means
   a. emanating.
   b. appeasing.
   c. attempting.
   d. fluctuating.

5. I was shocked when the family requested that I attend the funeral and give the
   a. tenet.
   b. eulogy.
   c. captions.
   d. litigations.

6. A quick score plunged the crowd into gloom, when just moments before their expectations had reached a
   a. restoration.
   b. transition.
   c. zenith.
   d. fruition.

7. The doctor used an ultrasound device to stimulate blood flow to the patient's ankle.
   Stimulate means to
   a. remove toxins and fight infection.
   b. create a digital image of the affected area.
   c. discourage development or decrease activity.
   d. encourage development or increase activity.

8. A person who is severe in manner or appearance is said to be
   a. affable.
   b. austere.
   c. jovial.
   d. morose.

9. Which word has almost the same meaning as **aversion**?
   a. Distraction
   b. Downturn
   c. Distaste
   d. Problem

10. A person who asserts authority in a domineering manner can be described as
    a. trivial.
    b. aloof.
    c. recalcitrant.
    d. officious.

11. The family tended to Roger's every need until he was satiated.
    Satiated means
    a. sleeping.
    b. satisfied.
    c. bored.
    d. jovial.

12. It's hard to discourage a person who is sanguine because they are
    a. tired.
    b. emotional.
    c. optimistic.
    d. depressed.

13. The hikers tried to delve briefly into the swamp but turned back.
    Delve means
    a. investigate.
    b. circumnavigate.
    c. go around.
    d. submerge.

14. The diner had the audacity to march into the kitchen and demand to see the chef.
    Audacity means
    a. impudence.
    b. destitution.
    c. garrulousness.
    d. firmament.

15. She was a fiery speaker who used catch phrases to foment enthusiasm in a crowd.
    Foment means
    a. stir up.
    b. garner.
    c. patronize.
    d. temporize.

16. The antique dealer had a penchant for shiny glass objects.
    Penchant means
    a. fondness.
    b. succor.
    c. diatribe.
    d. aversion.

READING COMPREHENSION: There are five reading passages in this section. Read each passage carefully. Then, on the basis of what you have read in the passage, select the best answer for each question.

PASSAGE 1

Ballast waifs are seeds that arrive on one shore from another in the soil placed in a ship's hold as ballast. One remarkably lovely and dreadfully damaging ballast waif is *Lythrum salicaria*, the bright purple, spiky flower known commonly as purple loosestrife. Purple loosestrife is not a newcomer to U.S. shores; it arrived from Eurasia, almost certainly via ship, some 200 years ago.

For all its beauty, purple loosestrife is a menace. The same long growing season that makes it so beloved by gardeners makes it a seed-making machine. A mature plant may produce two or three million seeds a year. It also propagates underground, sending out shoots and stems in all directions.

Scientists took little notice of purple loosestrife until some time in the 1930s, when a particular strain began colonizing along the St. Lawrence River, an area rife with the sort of wetlands purple loosestrife likes best. Purple loosestrife does not just propagate wildly; it also adapts easily to changes in environment. As it starts up in a new area, it quickly outcompetes native grasses, sedges, and other flowering plants, forming dense stands of purple loosestrife where once heterogeneous wetland meadows existed. This not only eradicates the native plants but also removes food sources for migratory birds and other animals.

In recent years, purple loosestrife has had a devastating impact on native cattails and wild rice. It has invaded and destroyed spawning areas for fish. In rural areas, it is beginning to move away from wetlands and adapt to drier areas, encroaching on agricultural lands. In urban areas, it is blocking pipes and drainage canals. It has moved steadily westward and is now found in all states but Florida.

Attempts to control purple loosestrife have been only partially successful. It has proved resistant to many herbicides, and it is impervious to burning, as its root-stock lies beneath the surface and can reproduce from there. It can be mowed down and plowed under, and then replaced with a less invasive plant. This is very labor-intensive in marshy areas that are substantially overgrown, but it may be the only way of eliminating the pest.

17. According to the passage, all of these are true *except*
    a. purple loosestrife propagates through an underground system.
    b. purple loosestrife is found in urban and rural settings.
    c. purple loosestrife is best eradicated through controlled burning.
    d. purple loosestrife is not native to North and South America.

18. Which of these would be the best title for the passage?
    a. Floral Invasion
    b. Gardener's Worst Nightmare
    c. Migrating Plants
    d. Controlling Pesky Plants

19. The author suggests that people enjoy growing purple loosestrife because it
    a. keeps out other weeds.
    b. makes millions of seeds.
    c. has a long growing season.
    d. reduces weevils and insects.

20. In the context of the third paragraph, the word **dense** is used to mean
    a. intense.
    b. opaque.
    c. complicated.
    d. concentrated.

21. According to the passage, where would purple loosestrife least easily thrive?
    a. Among swampy areas of northern New Jersey
    b. In the wetland meadows of eastern Michigan
    c. Along the inland waterways of North Carolina
    d. Above the tree line in the mountains of Utah

22. According to the author, purple loosestrife can be eradicated by being mowed down, plowed under, and planted with other species. Which of the following information, if true, would provide the least support for this argument?
    a. *Lythrum salicaria* has been removed from some gardens through the careful use of an Australian slug.
    b. Replanted meadows where purple loosestrife once grew are slowly being taken over by a new, hardier strain of *Lythrum salicaria*.
    c. Cattails are coming back to some New York swampland once devastated by the incursion of *Lythrum salicaria*.
    d. Chopping up the rootstock of *Lythrum salicaria* with a plow adds an unexpected bonus in the form of nitrogen-rich fertilizer.

PASSAGE 2

When most people think about taking a nap, they typically envision being down for the count for at least an hour or two. A German study, however, has shown that if you really want to refresh your brain, a six-minute cat nap will do it. Not only will you feel better afterwards, but your ability to learn and remember will have improved as well.

As described in a recent article in the *Journal of Sleep Research*, students at the University of Düsseldorf participated in experiments in which they had to memorize a list of words and then either take a nap or play a video game. The ones who napped consistently scored higher than those who stayed awake.

The study may help scientists learn more about what happens when people go to sleep. They already know that the brain undergoes a number of significant changes in the process. "There are dramatic shifts in brain chemistry and electrophysiology," said Dr. Matthew Tucker, a researcher at Harvard University School of Medicine and the Center for Sleep and Cognition. "For example, we know that levels of the transmitter acetylcholine go down. And we think that when acetylcholine gets to a low point, it should have an enhancing effect on memory."

Experts believe that sleeping is the brain's chance to decide which details and memories from the day need to be placed in permanent storage and which ones need to be thrown out. It has to do this because there is only so much room in the brain for information.

Of course, those catnaps may be wonderful, but they can never replace the value of a solid eight hours of sleep. As Dr. Olaf Lahl, the study's lead author, phrases it, "A regular sleep schedule still plays an important role in overall well-being and health."

23. What is the main idea of this passage?
   a. Everyone has to have eight hours of sleep each night.
   b. Brief naps are enough to help energize most people.
   c. There is a limited amount of room in the brain for storage.
   d. Memorizing lists of words is more difficult than you'd think.

24. Sleeping apparently helps with everything *except*
   a. fatigue.
   b. memory.
   c. learning.
   d. appetite.

25. What happens when the level of acetylcholine decreases in the brain?
   a. A person gets sleepy.
   b. A person learns more slowly.
   c. A person's memory improves.
   d. A person's fatigue fades away.

26. What is one of the primary purposes of sleep, according to this passage?
   a. To allow a person mentally to sort out important and unnecessary information
   b. To let a person experience dreams and work out emotional issues
   c. To ensure that a person stays healthy and resists illness at all times
   d. To allow a person to experience dramatic changes in overall brain chemistry

27. Which of the following statements best states the conclusion of the passage?
   a. German studies about sleep deprivation are becoming scientifically accepted.
   b. Brain chemistry undergoes significant changes during the different stages of sleep.
   c. A solid night's sleep is not necessary if a person takes several naps each day.
   d. According to a study, catnaps are much more effective than you might think.

28. What can you infer about the brain's need to sort information during learning as a result of this study?
     a. People learn better if their brains have less temporary information.
     b. People learn better if their brains have more permanent information.
     c. People's brains need an extended rest to sort through information learned.
     d. People's brains need video games to sort through information learned.

PASSAGE 3

The "food pyramid" is a visual representation of how the different food groups can be combined to form a healthy diet. Although it has been a vital part of dietary guidelines for years, the pyramid is constantly undergoing analysis and revision as additional studying is done in nutritional fields. Recently, the pyramid has undergone another change regarding the unique dietary needs of seniors.

According to an article published in the January 2008 issue of the *Journal of Nutrition*, modifications in the pyramid for older adults include an emphasis on fiber and calcium, as well as on vitamins D and B12. By incorporating these changes, the pyramid now indicates that the nutrients found in a person's routine daily consumption typically are not enough for seniors. Seniors need supplementation.

As people age, they tend to move less and thus need fewer calories to maintain their weight. Because seniors tend to eat a more limited amount, dietitians urge them to choose wisely. They are urged to eat nutrient-rich meals featuring such food as fruits, vegetables, low-fat dairy products, and high-fiber whole grains. Some experts recommend that older people purchase packaged versions of perishable items because such foods last longer than the fresh kind. For example, dried and frozen fruit have a much longer shelf life, as do frozen or canned vegetables. Having a supply of these foods in the cupboard means fewer trips to the grocery store and less risk of running out of nutritional snacks.

The newly designed pyramid also focuses on the importance for older people of ingesting adequate amounts of fluids on a daily basis. This helps ensure proper digestion and prevent any possibility of dehydration.

Finally, the revised pyramid includes information on incorporating exercise and other physical activities into the lives of older adults. Suggestions include swimming, walking, or simple yard work. Because recent reports have stated that obesity levels for people older than 70 years of age are climbing, performing some type of regular exercise is more essential than ever.

29. The best title for this selection is
     a. America's Seniors Need Exercise.
     b. A New Food Pyramid for Seniors.
     c. Finding Supplementation for Aging.
     d. Dietary Changes in Older Americans.

30. The purpose of updating the food pyramid as described in the passage is to
    a. change how seniors eat.
    b. increase food supplement sales.
    c. encourage people to eat more fruit.
    d. convince older people to start swimming.

31. The passage says that seniors should support their digestion by
    a. taking vitamin D.
    b. eating fewer calories.
    c. drinking adequate fluids.
    d. incorporating some exercise into their regular routine.

32. Dried or frozen fruit is often recommended by dietitians because it is
    a. delicious.
    b. easier to store.
    c. more nutritional than fresh fruit.
    d. known to have a much longer shelf life.

33. The reason that the author of the passage suggests exercise such as swimming, walking, and yard work is because those activities are
    a. ways to interact with other people.
    b. things that can be done alone.
    c. low impact in nature and relatively safe.
    d. useless for burning up calories.

34. The author's purpose in writing this passage was primarily to
    a. alert people to the different dietary needs of seniors.
    b. encourage students to study the pyramid's requirements.
    c. inform nurses about what supplements are most essential.
    d. educate physicians on the differences between dried and fresh fruit.

PASSAGE 4

Perhaps nothing mars the beauty and joy of a baby's arrival more than the presence of birth defects. Although the baby will certainly be just as welcomed and adored, these defects may affect these young new lives in unpleasant and even dangerous ways.

One of the best ways to prevent more than half of all possible birth defects to the brain and spine is extremely easy; women simply must make sure they are taking in enough folic acid before they conceive and then continue to do so throughout the course of their pregnancy. Folic acid is primarily responsible for making new cells, and during early gestation, the cells of the neural tube, which eventually becomes the infant's spinal cord and brain, are particularly demanding. Having adequate amounts of folic acid at this point ensures proper cell division and specialization. If there is not enough folic acid in the mother's body at this point, neural tube defects (NTDs) can occur in varying degrees of severity. One example of an NTD is spina bifida, a life-threatening situation; another is anencephaly, a fatal condition.

Experts recommend that women take 400 mcg of folic acid a day throughout their childbearing years. They can do this by taking daily multivitamin supplements that contain folic acid, by taking a single daily supplement of folic acid, or by adding fortified breakfast cereals to their daily menu. It is not adequate to wait until becoming pregnant to start supplementing with folic acid. The body must have a good supply before conception takes place. In addition, many women do not realize they are pregnant for several weeks. By the time they do realize it, and begin increasing their folic acid intake, the development phase for the embryo's brain and spinal cord has already passed.

In addition to causing NTDs, a lack of folic acid can also result in other health conditions, such as cleft lip and cleft palate. It can also raise the risk of Parkinson's disease. On the other hand, adequate amounts of folic acid can lower the risk of cardiovascular disease and cancers of the colon, cervix, and breast, as well as Alzheimer's disease.

35. The major subject of this passage is
    a. dealing with spina bifida.
    b. finding natural sources of folic acid.
    c. recognizing the symptoms of Parkinson's disease.
    d. understanding the importance of folic acid during gestation.

36. According to the passage, when should a woman start making sure she has an adequate supply of folic acid?
    a. The minute she finds out that she is pregnant
    b. Throughout her childbearing years
    c. During the second and third trimester of pregnancy
    d. Not before her obstetrician advises it

37. What conclusions can be drawn from the last sentence in the passage?
    a. Folic acid is not important after infancy.
    b. A good supply of folic acid prevents Alzheimer's disease.
    c. Folic acid plays an essential nutritional role throughout life.
    d. A lack of folic acid in adulthood can result in cleft palates and cleft lips.

38. All of the following are examples of conditions resulting from a lack of folic acid *except*
    a. cleft palate.
    b. spina bifida.
    c. anencephaly.
    d. breast cancer.

39. What does the words **mars** mean as used in this passage?
    a. Emphasizes
    b. Tarnishes
    c. Exemplifies
    d. Characterizes

40. The passage suggests that women can take folic acid in all of the following ways *except*
    a. as a topical shot.
    b. as a single supplement.
    c. as part of a multivitamin supplement.
    d. as part of fortified foods such as cereals.

PASSAGE 5

The Red List is published annually by the World Conservation Union to indicate to the world which species are threatened, endangered, and extinct. The most recent list included nearly 16,000 endangered species, including, incredibly, nearly every ape on the planet.

The Western Lowland gorilla moved from "endangered" to "critically endangered" in 2007. "Critically endangered" indicates that its population and range are shrinking, and it is in imminent danger of extinction. The Mountain gorilla, once studied by George Schaller and Dian Fossey in the 1960s, has also been endangered for years.

The gorilla has the misfortune to be native to an area that has been ravaged by war. Rwanda and the Congo are war-torn nations, and the resulting damage to habitat has affected gorillas as well as humans. Gorilla populations have also been ransacked by the Ebola virus, which has killed an estimated 90 percent of the gorilla population in each area of western and central Africa where it has been found.

Like humans, gorillas tend to have a single offspring at a time, with each one gestating for about nine months. Females do not mature until around age six, and nearly half of baby gorillas do not survive till breeding age.

The number-one threat to gorillas, however, is human greed. Humans are burning down the forests where the last remaining gorilla families live. They are doing this to harvest charcoal, which is used to fuel cooking fires throughout the region. In addition, they are poaching the last remaining gorillas for meat and their hands or other parts, which are considered a delicacy in Africa and are used medicinally in parts of Asia.

Even the tourist industry, once thought to be a way to preserve the ape population, has proved deadly to the gorillas. Many have died from measles or respiratory infections caught from humans. Despite the best efforts of dedicated conservationists and African rangers, some give these vegetarian cousins of *Homo sapiens* no more than a decade before all wild specimens are eradicated.

41. The author's tone indicates that she feels the eradication of apes is
    a. inevitable.
    b. shocking.
    c. intentional.
    d. impossible.

42. Based on information in the passage, about how many gorillas have survived in regions where the Ebola virus is prevalent?
    a. About 1 percent
    b. About 1 in 10
    c. About half
    d. Only 9 in 10

43. How are the ideas in the first two sentences of the second paragraph related?
    a. Sentence 2 provides a contrast to sentence 1.
    b. Sentence 2 is the next step after sentence 1.
    c. Sentence 2 defines a term that appears in sentence 1.
    d. Sentence 2 provides support for a theory in sentence 1.

44. The main point of the passage is that
    a. gorillas are not designed for survival.
    b. conservation is unrealistic.
    c. humans put gorillas at risk.
    d. we all must protect our ape cousins.

45. The author's purpose in the fifth paragraph is to
    a. introduce a hypothesis and support it with examples.
    b. compare some indignities perpetrated on apes.
    c. list some possible reasons for the extinction of species.
    d. contradict theories suggested in earlier paragraphs.

46. By the end of the passage, the author concludes that
    a. Africans care little about gorillas.
    b. the large apes should fight back.
    c. humans are largely evil.
    d. gorillas may not survive.

WORD KNOWLEDGE: Read each sentence carefully. Then, on the basis of what is stated in the sentence, select the answer to the incomplete statement. The answers will be found at the end of the test.

47. Compared to modern computers, yesterday's typewriters seem awfully
    a. urbane.
    b. intrepid.
    c. antediluvian.
    d. fulminating.

48. The patient's dirty clothes and unkempt appearance suggested to the doctor that he was living in squalid conditions.
    Squalid means
    a. filthy.
    b. luxurious.
    c. foreign.
    d. dangerous.

49. The new clerk hoped to find an older, more experienced colleague who could give her career advice and act as her
    a. mentor.
    b. attaché.
    c. delegate.
    d. misnomer.

50. Which of the following words is a synonym for **protocol**?
    a. Ideas
    b. Rules
    c. Preferences
    d. Obsessions

51. I did not write down the patient's comments word for word; instead I _____ them.
    a. emphasized
    b. underlined
    c. paraphrased
    d. imitated

52. Which of the following words means the opposite of **taciturn**?
    a. Aloof
    b. Generous
    c. Outgoing
    d. Puzzled

53. Dr. Parker was reluctant to say anything that might upset his patients.
    Reluctant means
    a. eager.
    b. anxious.
    c. happy.
    d. unwilling.

54. I was so nervous about my new job that I couldn't sleep, and I needed the sedative more than the patient did.
    Sedative refers to a medication that
    a. soothes or tranquilizes.
    b. promotes health.
    c. cures illness.
    d. stops infection.

55. I felt honored when the hospital asked me to give a testimonial for the great Doctor Edwards when she retired.
    Testimonial means
    a. dedication.
    b. requiem.
    c. rejoinder.
    d. praising speech.

56. If a patient's notes state that he is corpulent, it means that he is
    a. overweight.
    b. quite tall.
    c. elderly.
    d. masculine.

57. Someone who is able to tell the difference between a sensible idea and a fad can
    a. discriminate.
    b. discard.
    c. pretend.
    d. accuse.

58. After a series of sporadic achievements, Kevin gave up his dream of his own business.
    Sporadic means
    a. immodest.
    b. depleting.
    c. offensive.
    d. infrequent.

59. The airplane noise made it hard to sleep, and turbulence left them
    a. pacific.
    b. shuddering.
    c. somnambulant.
    d. verbatim.

60. His constant complaints without any apparent accompanying symptoms convinced the nurses that he was a
    a. litigant.
    b. collaborator.
    c. hypochondriac.
    d. neophyte.

Mathematics

45 Minutes

Work each problem carefully. Use scrap paper to do your calculations. The correct answers will be found at the end of the test.

1. How is $\dfrac{8}{2}$ expressed as a percentage?
   a. 4 percent
   b. 40 percent
   c. 400 percent
   d. 4,000 percent

2. $287 \times 36 =$
   a. 8,452
   b. 9,282
   c. 9,862
   d. 10,332

3. What is the prime number between 34 and 39?
   a. 35
   b. 36
   c. 37
   d. 38

4. If $3 + 4x = 23$, what is the value of x?
   a. 2
   b. 3
   c. 4
   d. 5

5. $1\dfrac{2}{3} + \dfrac{4}{5} =$
   a. $\dfrac{7}{15}$
   b. $\dfrac{13}{15}$
   c. $\dfrac{37}{15}$
   d. $\dfrac{52}{15}$

Use the information below to answer questions 6 and 7.

	Cases sold	Individual bottles sold	Total bottles
1997 Pinot Noir	5,437	15,229	80,473
1994 Pinot Gris	4,913	18,445	77,401
1992 Chardonnay	6,110	14,757	88,077
2001 Bordeaux	7,226	11,934	98,646

6. Which wine sold the most cases but the fewest individual bottles?
    a. 1997 Pinot Noir
    b. 1994 Pinot Gris
    c. 1992 Chardonnay
    d. 2001 Bordeaux

7. Which wine had the largest percentage of sales in individual bottles?
    a. 1997 Pinot Noir
    b. 1994 Pinot Gris
    c. 1992 Chardonnay
    d. 2001 Bordeaux

8. $7,259 - 3,687 =$
    a. 3,572
    b. 3,672
    c. 4,572
    d. 5,472

9. $5^{10} \div 5^2 =$
    a. 5^5
    b. 5^6
    c. 5^8
    d. 5^{12}

10. $3.902 \times 28 =$
    a. 1.09256
    b. 10.9256
    c. 109.256
    d. 1,092.56

11. What is 60 percent of 70?
    a. 35
    b. 42
    c. 46
    d. 54

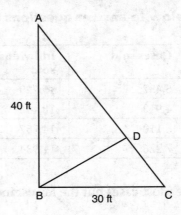

12. In the triangle ABC, BC is 30 feet and AB is 40 feet, what is the length of AC?
    a. 45 ft
    b. 50 ft
    c. 60 ft
    d. 70 ft

Use the following chart for questions 13–14.

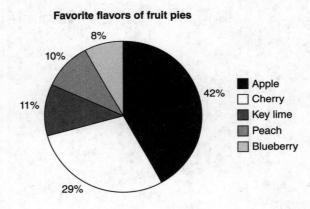

13. Which flavors of pies together are equal in popularity to cherry pie?
    a. Apple, key lime, peach
    b. Blueberry, peach, apple
    c. Key lime, peach
    d. Blueberry, peach, key lime

14. Which pies together are greater in popularity than apple?
    a. Key lime, cherry
    b. Blueberry, peach, key lime, cherry
    c. Peach, key lime, cherry
    d. Both B and C

15. If Jacob spends 45 minutes per day playing video games, how long does he play in one week?
    a. 3 hours, 45 minutes
    b. 4 hours
    c. 4 hours, 15 minutes
    d. 5 hours, 15 minutes

16. If a table measures 48 inches across, approximately how many centimeters is that?
    a. 20
    b. 50
    c. 60
    d. 120

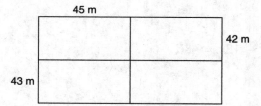

17. A rectangular field was divided into four plots, as shown above. The length was divided in half and the width was divided into slightly uneven plots. What is the area of the field?
    a. 3,825 meters
    b. 175 meters
    c. 1,890 meters
    d. 7,650 meters

18. $3 - 1\dfrac{5}{6} =$

    a. $\dfrac{1}{7}$

    b. $\dfrac{1}{6}$

    c. $\dfrac{6}{7}$

    d. $\dfrac{7}{6}$

19. What is the most reduced form of $2x^5y^3 + 4x^4y^6$?
    a. $x^4y^3(x + 2y^3)$
    b. $x^3y^4(x + 2y^3)$
    c. $2x^4y^3(x + 2y^3)$
    d. $4x^4y^3(x + 2y^3)$

20. If Bob is paid $5,000 less than the sum of Al and Carl's salaries, which of the following mathematical statements expresses this relationship?
    a. $B = A + C - 5,000$
    b. $B = A \times C - 5,000$
    c. $B = A + C + 5,000$
    d. $B = A \times C + 5,000$

21. What is the range of the data set shown below, which were the results of nine volume measurements of a solution during a lab?

    {2.4 mL, 3.2 mL, 3.7 mL, 3.7 mL, 4.5 mL, 6.5 mL, 7.3 mL, 8.1 mL, 12.2 mL}

    a. 3.7 mL
    b. 4.5 mL
    c. 5.8 mL
    d. 9.8 mL

22. Solve for x: $x^2 - 12x = -36$.
    a. 2
    b. 3
    c. 4
    d. 6

23. Solve for x: $x^3 - 64x = 0$.
    a. $x = 0, \pm 8$
    b. $x = 0, \pm 6$
    c. $x = 0, \pm 4$
    d. $x = 0, \pm 2$

24. Solve for x: $(4x - 1)^2 = 121$.
    a. -3
    b. 2
    c. 3
    d. 6

The three most commonly used temperature scales are Fahrenheit (°F), Celsius (°C), and Kelvin (K). They are based on the freezing point and boiling point of water as shown below.

Temperature scale	Freezing point of water	Boiling point of water
Fahrenheit (°F)	32	212
Celsius (°C)	0	100
Kelvin (K)	273	373

The formula for temperature conversion from Fahrenheit to Celsius is $°C \times \dfrac{9}{5} + 32$.

25. If the temperature of a patient was 40°C, what would her temperature be in Fahrenheit?
    a. 99.5°F
    b. 100°F
    c. 101.3°F
    d. 104°F

26. If it is 90°F, approximately what temperature is it on the Celsius scale?
    a. 18°C
    b. 32°C
    c. 58°C
    d. 104°C

27. A square room has an area of 196 ft². If the length and width of the room are the same, how wide is the room?
    a. 12 ft
    b. 13 ft
    c. 14 ft
    d. 16 ft

28. $3.98 \times 0.72 =$
    a. 3.26
    b. 2.8656
    c. 4.7
    d. 5.0293

29. The ratio of flour to sugar in a certain recipe is 3:2. If Don is making as much of the recipe as he can and he only has nine cups of flour, how much sugar will he use?
    a. 3
    b. 4.5
    c. 6
    d. 7.5

30. What is the sum of the prime factors of 30?

    a. 2

    b. 5

    c. 10

    d. 15

31. What is the average (mean) of 8, −4, 3, 9, and 4?

    a. 2.75

    b. 3

    c. 4

    d. 5.6

32. $2\dfrac{3}{4} \div \dfrac{7}{8} =$

    a. $\dfrac{15}{7}$

    b. $\dfrac{77}{32}$

    c. $\dfrac{22}{7}$

    d. $\dfrac{63}{16}$

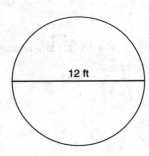

12 ft

33. What is the area of this circle?

    a. 12π ft²

    b. 18π ft²

    c. 24π ft²

    d. 36π ft²

34. $15,829 + 1,302 =$

    a. 16,131

    b. 17,031

    c. 17,131

    d. 18,131

35. Which of the following mathematical statements best reflects this graph?

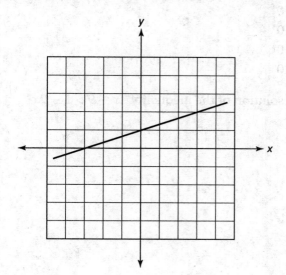

   a. $y = \dfrac{1}{3x} + 1$

   b. $y = \dfrac{1}{-3x} - 1$

   c. $y = 3x + 1$

   d. $y = 3x - 1$

36. $\dfrac{1}{3} \div \dfrac{5}{9} =$

   a. $\dfrac{3}{5}$

   b. $\dfrac{5}{3}$

   c. $\dfrac{5}{9}$

   d. $\dfrac{1}{9}$

37. What is the average of the numbers 24, 53, 70, 89, 34, and 30?
   a. 84
   b. 39
   c. 71
   d. 50

38. Express 239 in scientific notation.
   a. 2.39×10^0
   b. 2.39×10^1
   c. 2.39×10^2
   d. 2.39×10^3

39. $(-5.4 \times 10^7) \div (2.7 \times 10^3) =$
    a. -1.5×10^4
    b. -2.0×10^4
    c. -3.5×10^4
    d. -5.0×10^4

40. What is the solution of the inequality $3x - 9 > 1 - 2x$?
    a. $x > \dfrac{1}{2}$
    b. $x < \dfrac{1}{2}$
    c. $x > 2$
    d. $x < 2$

Science

45 Minutes

Read each question carefully and then select the correct answer. The correct answers will be found at the end of the test.

1. Light is shined on a plant from a fixed position. As the plant grows, it tends to bend toward the light. This tendency is called
   a. geotropism.
   b. hydrotropism.
   c. phototropism.
   d. auxinism.

2. A change in the _____ leads to a mutation of an organism.
   a. transfer RNA
   b. amino acid in a protein synthesis
   c. messenger RNA
   d. nitrogen base sequence in DNA

3. When a solute such as iodine is dissolved in _____, the solution is referred to as a tincture.
   a. water
   b. ether
   c. alcohol
   d. a base

4. A potassium ion (K^+) can be formed from a potassium atom (K) by
   a. losing a neutron.
   b. gaining a neutron.
   c. gaining an electron.
   d. losing an electron.

5. A short pea plant that is homozygous recessive for tallness (tt) is crossed with a tall pea plant which is heterozygous for tallness (Tt). The expected outcome is
   a. 25 percent of the plants will be short.
   b. 75 percent of the plants will be short.
   c. 50 percent of the plants will be tall.
   d. 100 percent of the plants will be tall.

6. A male who is color-blind (X′Y) produces offspring with a female carrier of the same disorder (X′X). Which of the following is expected? Use a chart like this for your answer.

	X′	Y
X′		
X		

a. All of the children will be color-blind.
b. None of the children will be color-blind.
c. The male offspring will be color-blind.
d. The offspring have a 50 percent chance of being color-blind.

7. Two organisms live in a symbiotic relationship from which both benefit. This is best described as
a. mutualism.
b. parasitism.
c. commensalism.
d. conservation.

8. Which of the following is *not* helpful in protecting the environment?
a. Recycling plastic, glass, and paper
b. Making use of solar energy
c. Burning fossil fuels
d. Driving hydrogen fuel-cell cars

9. Consider the following diagram:

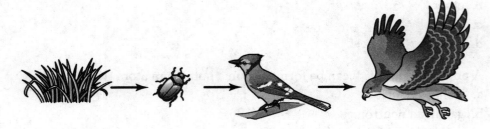

This diagram shows
a. a food web.
b. a food chain.
c. decomposers in action.
d. what happens when sunlight is not available.

10. If the rate of change in velocity of an airplane has a negative value, the airplane has
a. stopped.
b. slowed down.
c. crashed an hour ago.
d. maintained a constant speed.

11. A runner sprints at a constant speed of 4 meters per second. How far will the runner travel in 20 seconds?
    a. 5 meters
    b. 800 meters
    c. 120 meters
    d. 80 meters

12. To be isotopes, two atoms of the same element must have a different number of
    a. neutrons.
    b. protons.
    c. electrons.
    d. quarks.

13. Depending on its environment, a substance that can act as either an acid or a base is described as
    a. amphoteric.
    b. an isomer.
    c. hydrolytic.
    d. a polymer.

14. A certain substance is not broken down in a chemical reaction. The substance is most likely
    a. a compound.
    b. an aqueous solution.
    c. an element.
    d. a heterogeneous mixture.

15. A hydrogen ion concentration of 1×10^{-7} M in a solution is considered
    a. basic.
    b. alkali.
    c. acidic.
    d. neutral.

16. The radioactive isotope I-131 has a half-life of 8 days. What fraction of a sample of I-131 will remain after 24 days?
    a. $\dfrac{1}{4}$
    b. $\dfrac{1}{16}$
    c. $\dfrac{1}{8}$
    d. $\dfrac{1}{2}$

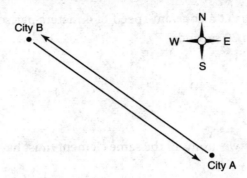

17. An airplane travels 500 miles northeast and then, on the return trip, travels 500 miles southwest. Which of the following is *true*?
    a. The displacement of the plane is 1,000 miles, and the distance traveled is 0 miles.
    b. The displacement of the plane is 1,000 miles, and the distance traveled is 1,000 miles.
    c. The displacement of the plane is 0 miles, and the distance traveled is 0 miles.
    d. The displacement of the plane is 0 miles, and the distance traveled is 1,000 miles.

18. The reaction $2NaI + Cl_2 \rightarrow 2NaCl + I_2$ demonstrates a
    a. decomposition reaction.
    b. synthesis reaction.
    c. single replacement reaction.
    d. double replacement reaction.

19. An electromagnet is holding a 1,500-kilogram car at a height of 25 meters above the ground. The magnet then experiences a power outage, and the car falls to the ground (without injuring anyone). Which of the following is *false*?
    a. The car had a potential energy of 367.5 kJ.
    b. 367.5 kJ of potential energy is converted to kinetic energy.
    c. The car still has a potential energy of 367.5 kJ when it hits the ground.
    d. The potential energy is converted to kinetic energy and then converted to sound energy.

20. What term describes the electrons in the outermost principal energy level of an atom?
    a. Vector
    b. Core
    c. Kernel
    d. Valence

21. In the presence of a base, blue litmus paper is
    a. clear.
    b. blue.
    c. pink.
    d. red.

22. Which compound below contains the alcohol functional group?
    a. $C_2H_5OCH_3$
    b. C_3H_4
    c. CH_3CH_2CHO
    d. C_3H_7OH

23. Blood with pH of 7.4 indicates that the blood sample is
    a. strongly acidic.
    b. strongly basic.
    c. weakly acidic.
    d. weakly basic.

24. Among the following elements, which is a nonmetal?
    a. Mercury
    b. Magnesium
    c. Sulfur
    d. Isomers

25. Two organic compounds have the same formula but different molecular structures. These compounds are said to be
    a. isofers.
    b. isocompounds.
    c. isotopes.
    d. isomers.

26. The radioactive isotope has a half-life of 20 years. How many grams of a 6-gram sample will remain after 40 years?
    a. 8 g
    b. 1.5 g
    c. 6 g
    d. 3 g

27. The human embryo develops in the female's
    a. menstrual cycle.
    b. uterus.
    c. vaginal canal.
    d. cervix.

28. Which of the following develops so that nutrients can reach the human embryo?
    a. Ovary
    b. Sperm
    c. Amnion
    d. Placenta

29. The small intestine has tiny structures designed for absorption. These are called
    a. villi.
    b. veins.
    c. venons.
    d. root tips.

30. Examples of biomes do *not* include
    a. deserts.
    b. tundra.
    c. tropical rainforests.
    d. neighborhoods in a city.

31. The scientific name for a house cat is *Felis catus*. This indicates the house cat's
    a. kingdom and family.
    b. order and subspecies.
    c. phylum and class.
    d. genus and species.

32. Which of the following statements is *false*?
    a. The exact age of a fossil can be determined by examining rock layers.
    b. Radioisotope dating can help determine the approximate age of a fossil.
    c. It is possible to determine the approximate age of a rock.
    d. Just a small number of organisms that ever lived on Earth are still alive today.

33. Natural selection does *not* include the idea that
    a. only the genes of the most fit organisms will be passed on.
    b. all organisms have a fair and equal chance of surviving.
    c. only the fittest organisms survive.
    d. there is a competition between organisms for survival.

34. Which of the following particles/rays is *not* a type of radioactive emanation?
    a. Alpha particle
    b. Beta particle
    c. Gamma ray
    d. Carbon-12

35. The strongest acid can be found in which of the following pH ranges?
    a. 11.1–12
    b. 7.1–8.2
    c. 4.5–5.7
    d. 1.0–2.0

36. The symbol K on the periodic table stands for
    a. potassium.
    b. calcium.
    c. carbon.
    d. phosphorus.

37. Which of the following reactions releases heat energy?
    a. Double replacement
    b. Decomposition
    c. Endothermic
    d. Exothermic

38. Which gas law states that the volume of a gas is inversely proportional to the pressure?
    a. Ideal gas law
    b. Boyle's law
    c. Combined gas law
    d. Charles' law

39. What type of bond is created when bromine and magnesium are reacted to form $MgBr_2$?
    a. Polar covalent
    b. Metallic
    c. Ionic
    d. Nonpolar covalent

40. When one liquid evaporates much faster than another liquid, the first liquid is said to be more
    a. volatile.
    b. transient.
    c. viscous.
    d. evaporative.

41. Which compound is nonpolar and contains a nonpolar covalent bond?
    a. F_2
    b. HI
    c. KCl
    d. NH_3

42. When solid iodine becomes gaseous iodine with no apparent liquid phase in between, the process is called
    a. evaporation.
    b. condensation.
    c. sublimation.
    d. precipitation.

43. What area of the periodic table shows the most nonmetallic elements?
    a. Upper left
    b. Upper right
    c. Lower left
    d. Lower right

44. Diamond and graphite are allotropes of
    a. oxygen.
    b. carbon.
    c. hydrogen.
    d. water.

45. What is the coefficient of O_2 after the following equation is balanced? $\_CH_4 + \_O_2 \rightarrow \_CO_2 + \_H_2O$.
    a. 1
    b. 2
    c. 3
    d. 4

46. Within the human kidney, which of the following works to filter the blood?
    a. Nephron
    b. Urethra
    c. Neutron
    d. Epiglottis

47. When there are no cone cells in an animal's retina, that animal most likely cannot
    a. determine various shades of colors.
    b. move the eyeball.
    c. focus properly.
    d. close its eyelid.

48. Of the following organisms, which is an invertebrate?
    a. Starfish
    b. Cat
    c. Human
    d. Mouse

49. Across which of the following does gas exchange take place?
    a. Skin
    b. Nasal cavity
    c. Capillaries
    d. Bronchioles

50. Which chamber of the heart receives blood from the lungs?
    a. Left atrium
    b. Right atrium
    c. Left ventricle
    d. Right ventricle

51. The space where a nervous impulse passes from one neuron to another is called the
    a. gap.
    b. neurotransmitter.
    c. synapse.
    d. sodium pump.

52. The number 1,000,000 is what power of 10?
    a. 10^{-6}
    b. 10^6
    c. 1^6
    d. 0.000001

53. The quantity 6,180 meters can be rewritten as
    a. 6.180×10^3 m.
    b. 6,180 km.
    c. $6,180 \times 10^3$ m.
    d. 180×103 m.

54. How many millimeters are there in one centimeter?
    a. 10,000
    b. 1,000
    c. 100
    d. 10

55. Which isotope below contains the greatest number of neutrons?
    a. $^{35}_{17}Cl$
    b. $^{18}_{8}O$
    c. $^{40}_{18}Ar$
    d. $^{41}_{20}Ca$

56. Aluminum (Al) has 13 protons in its nucleus. What is the number of electrons in an Al^{3+} ion?
    a. 13
    b. 10
    c. 16
    d. 3

57. How many electrons can be held in the third PEL of an atom?
    a. 2
    b. 8
    c. 18
    d. 32

58. Which of the following wavelengths of visible light is best absorbed by chlorophyll?
    a. 300 nm
    b. 495 nm
    c. 665 nm
    d. 550 nm

59. The xylem vessels of a plant are responsible for carrying
    a. water up through the plant.
    b. light energy to the leaves.
    c. chlorophyll to the leaves.
    d. oxygen into the leaves.

60. When placed in distilled water, a human red blood cell
    a. shrivels up.
    b. neither shrinks nor swells.
    c. takes up more salts to balance all concentrations.
    d. swells to a larger size.

Practice Test 5

Verbal Ability

Word Knowledge and Reading Comprehension

45 minutes

WORD KNOWLEDGE: Read each sentence carefully. Then, on the basis of what is stated in the sentence, select the answer to the incomplete statement. The answers will be found at the end of the test.

1. One of the thieves implicated his friend in the break-in.
   Implicated means
   a. complimented.
   b. informed on.
   c. prevaricated.
   d. palpitated.

2. Her assistants said she was hard to work for because she was so
   a. amorous.
   b. lenient.
   c. wistful.
   d. fastidious.

3. The rumor campaign began as gossip but soon became
   a. insidious.
   b. introverted.
   c exorbitant.
   d. indignant.

4. When the invading army seized the town, the general issued a series of
   a. analyses.
   b. edicts.
   c. queries.
   d. invoices.

5. After the ill-fated party, there remained a vast schism between the families.
    Schism means
    a. compact.
    b. mystery.
    c. crevasse.
    d. relationship.

6. The new salesman tried to succeed in the big city, but his manners seemed
    a. provincial.
    b. blatant.
    c. intimate.
    d. spurious.

7. The new player threw down the gauntlet by demanding the ball in tight games.
    To **throw down a gauntlet** means to
    a. fall into a reverie.
    b. put on a disguise.
    c. issue an epithet.
    d. offer a challenge.

8. If you simply invert the pump, the vapor lock will clear and reset.
    Invert means to
    a. shake thoroughly.
    b. turn upside down.
    c. twist from side to side.
    d. lay down flat.

9. After hiring the most qualified but obnoxious people, she hired someone skilled
    but more
    a. amiable.
    b. belligerent.
    c. prestigious.
    d. ostensible.

10. After testing the chunk of gold and realizing that it was fake, he felt
    a. exonerated.
    b. magnanimous.
    c. hoodwinked.
    d. benign.

11. A person who worries that something bad is about to happen is said to be
    a. apprehensive.
    b. menial.
    c. laconic.
    d. protean.

12. Which word has almost the same meaning as **sanction**?
    a. Define
    b. Inform
    c. Authorize
    d. Palpitate

13. A patient who is greatly depressed can be described as
    a. morose.
    b. placid.
    c. literal.
    d. profane.

14. The credulous patient believed the stories he read about treatments that produced miracle cures.
    Credulous means
    a. naive.
    b. skeptical.
    c. knowledgeable.
    d. confused.

15. A person who is orderly
    a. puts things away.
    b. leaves the house.
    c. makes a mistake.
    d. asks for help.

16. The three doctors decided to collaborate on the project. This means that they are going to
    a. start over again.
    b. work as a team.
    c. stop work temporarily.
    d. work harder.

READING COMPREHENSION: There are five reading passages in this section. Read each passage carefully. Then, on the basis of what you have read in the passage, select the best answer for each question.

PASSAGE 1

Elk were once found in the East, from Georgia north to New York and Connecticut. By the time of the Civil War, hunting and habitat destruction had caused their extinction in most eastern states. All of the eastern subspecies are now extinct. Elk County, Pennsylvania, was without elk for over a century.

At the beginning of the twentieth century, herds of elk in the Rocky Mountains faced death by starvation as encroaching farms depleted their winter-feeding grounds, and finally the government decided to intercede. They gathered up elk from Yellowstone National Park and shipped 50 of them to Pennsylvania.

At that early date, 1913, there was little understanding of the kind of acclimatization required when moving large animals from one habitat to another. The elk were released from cattle cars and chased into the wild to fend for themselves. Two years later, 95 more elk were moved from Yellowstone to Pennsylvania.

The elk tended to move toward farming areas because that was where the food was. Although they were protected, their destruction of farmland caused farmers to poach them illegally. In a 1971 survey, researchers found about 65 animals. Intensive work by the Bureau of Forestry to improve elk habitat, especially through reclamation of old strip mines, brought those numbers up to 135 by the early 1980s. By the year 2000, there were over 500 elk in Pennsylvania, including many in Elk County.

In 1984, hunters established the Rocky Mountain Elk Foundation, whose mission is to reintroduce elk in the states where they once roamed. At present, new herds are established in Arkansas, Kentucky, Michigan, and Wisconsin, in addition to Pennsylvania. There is talk of moving herds to Tennessee and to the Adirondack range in New York. It seems fairly clear that improving habitat for elk reintroduction improves conditions for other wildlife—wild turkey, whitetail deer, and black bear, among others.

Unlike in the 1910s, today reintroduction is vastly improved—far more closely monitored and controlled. Animals are checked for disease. Land trusts are used to preserve habitat and to keep the elk from moving too close to cropland.

17. According to this passage, a major early threat to elk populations was
    a. wolves and cougars.
    b. vehicular traffic.
    c. disease.
    d. hunting.

18. Based on information in the passage, about how many elk were moved from Yellowstone to Pennsylvania in the mid-1910s?
    a. 65
    b. 95
    c. 135
    d. 145

19. According to the passage, where might you see elk today?
    a. The Tennessee Valley
    b. Georgia
    c. The Adirondacks
    d. Arkansas

20. According to the passage, what is true of the elk in Pennsylvania today?
    a. They are the same as the elk who lived there 200 years ago.
    b. They are a different subspecies from the old Pennsylvania elk.
    c. They are a different subspecies from the elk found in the Rockies.
    d. They are only distantly related to the elk found in Yellowstone.

21. The passage implies that
    a. reclamation of land is a bad idea.
    b. hunters have ulterior motives for reintroducing elk.
    c. species reintroduction has improved over time.
    d. elk reintroduction may be doomed to failure.

22. Which of the following findings *best* supports the author's contention that elk repopulation is carefully monitored?
    a. Farming to raise deer, elk, and reindeer is increasingly popular.
    b. Before 1997, there had not been a wild elk in Kentucky in 150 years.
    c. Rocky Mountain elk were among the original animals at the Hearst Zoo.
    d. Jackson County is testing potential elk herds for chronic wasting disease.

PASSAGE 2

The health risks of coffee have long been debated, but a recent study has added another argument against too much coffee consumption. This study looked at the effect of drinking coffee on pregnant women. Conducted by physicians at Kaiser Permanente, the study explored the connection between caffeine and the risk of miscarriage.

The connection is one that has been explored before, but this study took a different approach. It took morning sickness into account, whereas other studies did not. The findings were significant: 200 milligrams of caffeine a day—about what is found in two cups of coffee—is enough to increase the risk of having a miscarriage. The source of the caffeine, whether coffee, tea, or soda, was irrelevant; the amount was the key.

This study followed more than 1,000 women who became pregnant within a two-year period. The amount of caffeine they drank was logged, as well as which women experienced a miscarriage. The results, as published in the January 2009 issue of the *American Journal of Obstetrics and Gynecology*, stated that the risk of miscarriage more than doubled in women who consumed 200 milligrams or more of caffeine per day.

Why does caffeine carry this risk? Researchers are not sure, but they theorize that the caffeine restricts blood flow to the placenta. This, in turn, can harm the developing fetus.

Does this mean physicians will start advising women to quit drinking coffee while pregnant? Yes and no. Some doctors will certainly take this report to heart and encourage their patients to stay away from more than one cup of coffee a day, just as they recommend not drinking alcohol or smoking cigarettes. Others are not so convinced and doubt that this single study is enough to overturn the established guidelines of the American College of Obstetricians and Gynecologists. Instead, they believe that a lot more research needs to be done.

23. What is the main idea of this passage?
    a. Coffee carries some obvious health risks for people.
    b. Two cups of coffee a day may be enough to raise the risk of miscarriage.
    d. There is a link between miscarriages and morning sickness.
    d. Miscarriage rates are on the rise internationally.

24. Based on the study, which aspect of caffeine consumption seemed to be the key to the risk of miscarriage?
    a. The source of the caffeine
    b. The time the caffeine is ingested
    c. The amount of caffeine ingested
    d. The time between doses of caffeine

25. What do some researchers believe is the link between caffeine and miscarriages?
    a. They think that caffeine inhibits placental blood flow.
    b. They believe that caffeine makes the heart beat too rapidly.
    c. They suspect that caffeine interferes with the immune system.
    d. They theorize that caffeine prevents some nutrients from crossing the placenta.

26. The word **overturn** as used in the last paragraph of the passage can best be defined as
    a. justify.
    b. invalidate.
    c. support.
    d. review.

27. Based on this passage, what conclusion can best be drawn about the advice physicians will give their pregnant patients about coffee consumption?
    a. Almost all of them will advise women to stop drinking any caffeine until after the baby is born.
    b. The majority will ignore the study altogether and continue to advise caffeine in moderation as before.
    c. All of them will demand additional research to be done before they change what they tell their patients.
    d. Some will continue to make their normal recommendations about caffeine, while others will be more cautious than before.

28. Based on this passage, what conclusion can best be drawn about the potential effects of drinking coffee?
    a. It is completely safe for anyone.
    b. There can be absolutely no concerns unless you are pregnant.
    c. It can be extremely dangerous for everyone.
    d. It may pose health risks for some people.

PASSAGE 3

Years of research have proven that Alzheimer's disease, along with other types of dementia, elevates the risk of dying early in the majority of patients. In a recent study performed by the Institute of Public Health at the University of Cambridge, scientists set out to determine just exactly how long people were likely to survive following the onset of dementia.

Currently, approximately 24 million people throughout the world suffer from the memory loss and orientation confusion that comes with Alzheimer's disease and other forms of dementia. That number appears to double every 20 years, and experts predict that by the year 2040, there will be 81 million people living with some level of the condition. The more the researchers and doctors can learn about what causes the problem, as well as how to treat it, the better prepared they will be to handle these millions of future patients.

To determine how people's life spans are affected by this medical condition, the scientists studied 13,000 seniors for a period of 14 years. During that time, 438 people developed dementia, the vast majority of whom died. The factors of age, disability, and gender were analyzed to see how they affected longevity as well.

Conclusions from the study showed that women tended to live slightly longer than men, averaging 4.6 years from the onset of dementia, as opposed to 4.1 years for men. The patients who were already weak or frail at the onset of the dementia died first, regardless of age. Marital status, living environment, and degree of mental decline, although relevant factors, were not shown to be influential.

Researchers from the University of Cambridge hope that this new information will help patients, clinicians, care providers, service providers, policy makers, and others who deal with dementia. The more they know, the better they will be able to respond to this heartbreaking condition.

29. The best title for this selection is
    a. Alzheimer's Disease on the Rise.
    b. Women's Life Spans Are Longer.
    c. Average Time of Survival with Dementia.
    d. The Effect of Marital Status on Longevity.

30. What fact did researchers already know before beginning this new study?
    a. Women with Alzheimer's disease tend to live slightly longer than their male counterparts.
    b. A patient's overall condition before dementia onset was a key factor in survival.
    c. People diagnosed with some kind of dementia usually have a higher risk of dying early.
    d. The living environment had a small influence on the overall life span of a patient with dementia.

31. The author mentions the number of patients with Alzheimer's disease to
    a. point out the rarity of the disease.
    b. emphasize the average age at which onset occurs.
    c. clarify why the disease strikes one sex more than another.
    d. explain why knowing more about the condition is so essential.

32. Why did the researchers undertake this new study on dementia?
    a. To better understand the effects of the disease.
    b. To educate families on how to cope with the condition.
    c. To show physicians and other professions a new kind of treatment.
    d. To prove that degree of mental decline is not the most important factor.

33. According to the passage, the factor that affects dementia survival rate the most is
    a. marital status.
    b. health at onset.
    c. living environment.
    d. degree of mental decline.

34. Ironically, the one group of people mentioned in the passage who will be unable to make use of the conclusions of the study are
    a. physicians.
    b. nurses.
    c. patients.
    d. policy makers.

PASSAGE 4

What do pilots, astronauts, physicians, and risk managers have in common? In this case, they are all part of an organization based in Memphis, Tennessee, called Lifewings Partners. This unusual group focuses on finding ways to eliminate mistakes made accidentally in medical settings within the United States.

Lifewings Partners emphasizes the need for a watchdog in various medical settings. According to the National Institutes of Health, approximately 98,000 patients die each year in U.S. health care settings due to nothing more than medical error. Some other experts suspect that the number is much higher, reaching as high as 145,000.

Examples include the man who had the wrong testicle removed in a Los Angeles hospital, a young boy who went in for a typical hernia surgery and ended up with brain damage from the anesthesia, and a hospital in Rhode Island that performed brain surgery on the wrong side of the brain—three times on three different patients in less than a year.

Since Lifewings Partners began seven years ago, more than 70 medical facilities have used their services. The company centers on ways to improve patient safety in much the same way pilots work to keep their passengers safe while in the air. They do this through a five-step program that requires hospitals to change their medical and communication procedures, train their doctors and nurses, and establish checklists and measurements designed to track outcomes.

In addition to making internal changes in medical settings, Lifewings Partners also works to educate patients on safety before they even enter the hospital. The company suggests that all consumers do the following: go online to obtain public information on a hospital's safety, talk to their doctors to see what safety standards are in place already, and ask professionals about which facilities tend to have the best safety records. As Steven Harden, founder and CEO of the organization, phrases it, "Just because a hospital has a great reputation for cutting-edge medicine doesn't necessarily mean the hospital is the safest place to for routine procedures." After all, some mistakes are too big and too irrevocable to risk.

35. What is the main emphasis in this passage?
    a. Medical mistakes are made in health centers every day.
    b. Lifewings Partners is made up of an eclectic mix of people.
    c. Lifewings Partners is working hard to prevent medical errors.
    d. Consumers should talk to their doctors about hospital safety.

36. Which detail from the passage best supports the idea that some medical settings can be dangerous to patients?
    a. A young boy went into a hospital for a hernia operation and ended up with brain damage.
    b. More than 70 medical facilities are currently suing Lifewings Partners' services.
    c. Lifewings Partners includes pilots, astronauts, doctors, and even risk managers.
    d. Experts suspect that more medical mistakes are made than are actually reported to the National Institutes of Health.

37. Which of the following is a step that Lifewings Partners requires its client hospitals to implement?
    a. Investigate the medical credentials of staff doctors and nurses.
    b. Prescreen patents for medical conditions.
    c. Enforce new rules regarding patients' health insurance.
    d. Establish measurements designed to track patient outcomes.

38. Which of the following is a conclusion that can be drawn from the last paragraph of the passage?
    a. Procedures that Lifewings Partners recommends are always effective.
    b. Medical mistakes can happen at even the best hospitals.
    c. Some hospitals know more about cutting-edge medicine than others.
    d. Medical mistakes will one day be completely eradicated.

39. The word **watchdog** as used in the second paragraph of the passage can best be defined as
    a. companion.
    b. guard.
    c. manager.
    d. punisher.

40. On which group of people does Lifewings Partners focus education efforts?
    a. Students
    b. CEOs
    c. Patients
    d. Pilots

PASSAGE 5

For years, anecdotal evidence from around the world indicated that amphibians were under siege, especially in the Caribbean. Finally, proof of this hypothesis is available, thanks to the concerted, Internet-based effort of scientists involved with the Global Amphibian Assessment.

Amphibians have a unique vulnerability to environmental changes thanks to their permeable skin and their need of specific habitats to allow their metamorphosis from larva to adult. Studies indicate that they are at risk due to global climate change, reduction in the ozone layer leading to an increased exposure to ultraviolet rays, interference with migratory pathways, drainage of wetlands, pollution by pesticides, erosion and sedimentation, and exposure to unknown pathogens thanks to the introduction of nonnative species. In other words, human progress is responsible for the losses this population is suffering.

Scientists have long considered amphibians a barometer of environmental health. In areas where amphibians are declining precipitously, environmental degradation is thought to be a major cause. Amphibians are not adaptable. They must have clean water in which to lay their eggs. They must have clean air to breathe after they grow to adulthood. Their "double life" as aquatic and land-dwelling animals means that they are at risk of a double dose of pollutants and other hazards.

The Global Amphibian Assessment concluded that nearly one-third of the world's amphibian species are under immediate threat of extinction. Nearly half of all species are declining in population. The largest numbers of threatened species are in Colombia, Mexico, and Ecuador, but the highest percentages of threatened species are in the Caribbean. In Haiti, for example, nine out of ten species of amphibians are threatened. In Jamaica, it is eight out of ten, and in Puerto Rico, seven out of ten.

Certainly, this is a disaster for amphibians, but scientists rush to point out that it may be equally a disaster for the rest of us on Earth. Even recent pandemics among amphibians may be caused by global changes. True, amphibians are ultrasensitive to such changes, but can reptiles, fish, birds, and mammals be far behind?

41. The main point of the passage is that
    a. the extinction of amphibians is due to global warming.
    b. amphibians really are barometers of environmental health.
    c. only equatorial amphibians are currently under siege.
    d. amphibians' "double life" on land and in water may end up saving them.

42. The passage implies that the Global Amphibian Assessment has done science a favor by
    a. setting forth a hypothesis that connects the environment to species' decline.
    b. eliminating the need to study the connection between extinction and environment.
    c. refuting a contention that had existed purely through anecdotal evidence.
    d. collecting data to prove something that was previously just a hypothesis.

43. The author's point in the first paragraph that amphibians are especially at risk in the Caribbean is *best* supported by evidence presented in which paragraph?
    a. 2
    b. 3
    c. 4
    d. 5

44. The author's purpose in the third paragraph is to
    a. provide background on the Assessment study.
    b. explain why amphibians are especially vulnerable.
    c. list types of amphibians that are most at risk.
    d. present examples of dangers from around the world.

45. What evidence could the author have included that would *best* support the main idea?
    a. Statistics involving numbers of frog species in Haiti
    b. Personal observations about the hazards of pollution
    c. Names of people involved in the Assessment study
    d. Comparisons between amphibians and reptiles

46. What can you infer from the author's mention of reptiles, birds, fish, and mammals at the end of the passage?
    a. These animals are less susceptible to climate change.
    b. These animals are even more sensitive to climate change.
    c. Climate change will eventually affect all animals, including humans.
    d. Climate change will only affect certain animals, not humans.

WORD KNOWLEDGE: Read each sentence carefully. Then, on the basis of what is stated in the sentence, select the answer to the incomplete statement. The answers will be found at the end of the test.

47. The angry people in the waiting room, tired of waiting for news about the patient, began **haranguing** the nurse
    a. lecturing the nurse.
    b. praising the nurse.
    c. looking for the nurse.
    d. questioning the nurse.

48. Breathing is achieved by altering the size of the chest cavity through movement of the diaphragm.
    Achieved means
    a. sponsored.
    b. indicated.
    c. accomplished.
    d. amplified.

49. When chemists in a laboratory want to make a reaction, they chose a
    a. catalyst.
    b. reactant.
    c. enabler.
    d. magnifier.

50. A person who behaves with cordial kindness is said to be
    a. affable.
    b. acrimonious.
    c. erudite.
    d. boorish.

51. Tired of working for free, Teddy took a summer job that paid a(n)
    a. schism.
    b. abacus.
    c. escarpment.
    d. stipend.

52. Everyone wanted to believe the investor's claims, yet he was a charlatan.
    Charlatan means
    a. imposter.
    b. bon mot.
    c. savant.
    d. comptroller.

53. The principal was known as a vivacious educator who was always
    a. latent.
    b. obdurate.
    c. contrite.
    d. animated.

54. A section of forest that is undeveloped or unexplored is said to be
    a. adroit.
    b. pristine.
    c. scrupulous.
    d. trenchant.

55. A trespass on forbidden ground is called a(n)
    a. incursion.
    b. shyster.
    c. resilience.
    d. omission.

56. Maureen looked haggard as she came back from the mountain hike.
    Haggard means
    a. excited and charged.
    b. wounded and limping.
    c. tired and worn.
    d. directed and purposeful.

57. The tales of the team's exploits turned out to be ephemeral and
    a. dissipating.
    b. legendary.
    c. renowned.
    d. heretical.

58. Our club's leader was famous for his Machiavellian maneuvers to retain his hold
    on power.
    Machiavellian means
    a. obstinate.
    b. cunning.
    c. cumbersome.
    d. incongruous.

59. The workers added reinforcing rods, but this only exacerbated the problem.
    Exacerbated means
    a. expunged.
    b. accrued.
    c. placated.
    d. aggravated.

60. The traffic cop was popular with commuters because he always had a jocund look on his face as he worked. He looked
    a. merry.
    b. cryptic.
    c. limpid.
    d. assiduous.

Mathematics

45 Minutes

Work each problem carefully. Use scrap paper to do your calculations. The correct answers will be found at the end of the test.

1. Given the equation $\dfrac{56}{(4x+8)} = \dfrac{1}{8}$, what is the value of x?
    a. 64
    b. 110
    c. 164
    d. 215

2. Find the roots of the quadratic equation $x^2 - 2x - 1 = 0$.
    a. $x = 1 \pm \sqrt{2}$
    b. $x = 1 \pm 2$
    c. $x = \sqrt{2} \pm 1$
    d. $x = 1 \pm \sqrt{3}$

3. $\left(\dfrac{4}{3}\right)^2 + \left(\dfrac{2}{4}\right)^2 =$

    a. $\dfrac{96}{36}$

    b. $\dfrac{84}{36}$

    c. $\dfrac{73}{36}$

    d. $\dfrac{65}{36}$

4. If $\dfrac{x}{y} = 8$ and $x = 64$, then what is the sum of x and y?
    a. 56
    b. 64
    c. 72
    d. 81

5.   On a single roll of a die, what is the probability of not getting a 2?

   a. $\dfrac{1}{6}$

   b. $\dfrac{1}{6}$

   c. $\dfrac{4}{6}$

   d. $\dfrac{5}{6}$

6.   What is the probability of randomly selecting a 10 card from a standard deck of cards?

   a. $\dfrac{1}{52}$

   b. $\dfrac{1}{13}$

   c. $\dfrac{12}{13}$

   d. $\dfrac{51}{52}$

7.   The number 8 is what percent of 5?
   a. 62.5 percent
   b. 160 percent
   c. 162.5 percent
   d. 200 percent

8. $294 \times 35 =$
   a. 2,352
   b. 10,290
   c. 12,520
   d. 14,009

9. Of the following numbers, which one is the only prime?
   a. 18
   b. 19
   c. 21
   d. 25

10. Which of the following expresses 65 percent as a decimal?
    a. 0.065
    b. 0.65
    c. 6.5
    d. 65

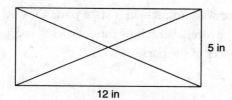

11. What is the measurement of one of the diagonals of this rectangle?
    a. 10 in
    b. 13 in
    c. 17 in
    d. 26 in

12. After taking inventory at his grocery store, Harry realizes that 20 percent of the items in stock are in the produce category. If he were to represent this in a pie chart, what would be the degree measure of the central angle that represents this percentage?
    a. 18°
    b. 20°
    c. 64°
    d. 72°

13. Polly's scores on the first four tests in her English class were 94, 91, 88, and 95. If all the tests counted equally, what was the average of her scores on those four tests?
    a. 90
    b. 91
    c. 92
    d. 93

14. Which of the following expressions is the mathematical equivalent of $7^3 \times 7^5$?
    a. 7^{-2}
    b. 7^2
    c. 7^8
    d. 7^{15}

15. A recent census of wild animals in a state park showed that there was a ratio of 15:8 raccoons to coyotes. Which of the following is a possible actual number of raccoons and coyotes in the park?
    a. 600:320
    b. 300:180
    c. 600:400
    d. 450:20

16. What is the mean (average) of 3, 14, 10, and −7?
    a. 4.5
    b. 5
    c. 7
    d. 8.5

17. Which of the following is the greatest prime number less than 30?
    a. 26
    b. 27
    c. 28
    d. 29

18. Which of the following has the largest value?
    a. $|-5.5|$
    b. −5.5
    c. −7.2
    d. $|-7.2|$

Use the line graph to answer questions 19–20.

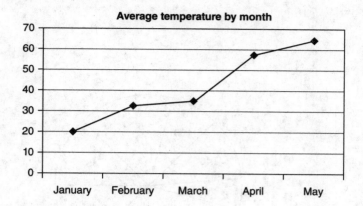

19. In the above chart, which month showed the smallest increase in temperature from the month before?
    a. February
    b. March
    d. April
    d. May

20. How many months show an increase of more than 10 degrees?
    a. 1
    b. 2
    c. 3
    d. 4

21 1,296 − 938 =
    a. 258
    b. 358
    c. 398
    d. 428

22. What is the probability of selecting a face card of a spade suit from two standard decks of cards?

    a. $\dfrac{3}{52}$

    b. $\dfrac{6}{52}$

    c. $\dfrac{6}{104}$

    d. $\dfrac{46}{104}$

23. What is the smallest prime number greater than 45?
    a. 46
    b. 47
    c. 48
    d. 49

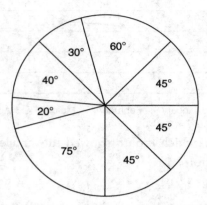

24. Approximately what percentage of the circle are the arcs of 40° and 20°?
    a. 6 percent
    b. 17 percent
    c. 30 percent
    d. 60 percent

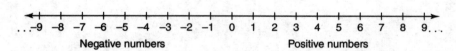

25. Which of these numbers could be shown on this number line in its exact location?
    a. π
    b. $\sqrt{7}$
    c. $\dfrac{9}{4}$
    d. $-3.1666...$

26. Which of the following expressions is the most simplified form of $\sqrt{56}$?
    a. $2\sqrt{7}$
    b. $2\sqrt{14}$
    c. $4\sqrt{7}$
    d. $4\sqrt{14}$

Sales by region

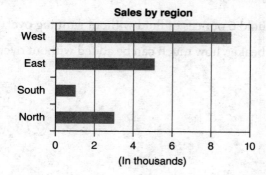

(In thousands)

27. What conclusion could a hospital administrator draw from this chart?
    a. About the same number of patients came from North and South.
    b. South was too far from the emergency room.
    c. East and West were about the same distance away.
    d. More patients came from West than all other regions.

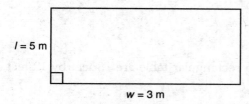

$l = 5$ m

$w = 3$ m

28. What is the perimeter of the rectangle above?
    a. 15 m
    b. 15 m²
    c. 16 m
    d. 16 m²

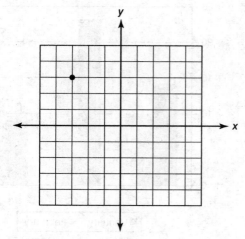

29. What are the coordinates of the point plotted above?
    a. (3, 3)
    b. (−3, −3)
    c. (3, −3)
    d. (−3, 3)

30. A beaker can hold 6 ounces of fluid without running over. If there is $2\frac{4}{5}$ ounces already in the beaker, how much can be added without overflowing the beaker?

   a. $4\frac{1}{5}$

   b. $3\frac{4}{5}$

   c. $2\frac{3}{5}$

   d. $3\frac{1}{5}$

31. 45 is 125% of what number?
   a. 24
   b. 25
   c. 30
   d. 36

32. If the sides of a rectangular table are 18 feet by 12 feet, what is the area of the table's surface?
   a. 96 ft²
   b. 144 ft²
   c. 216 ft²
   d. 256 ft²

Use the bar graph to answer questions 33–34.

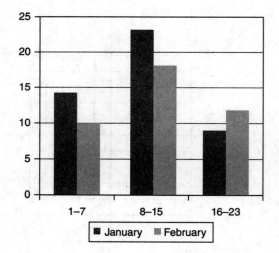

33. What is the best approximation of the number of patients ages 8–15 in both months combined?

    a. 18
    b. 23
    c. 40
    d. 46

34. Approximately how many more patients ages 1–7 than patients 16–23 were treated in January?

    a. 5
    b. 9
    c. 12
    d. 14

35. Solve for x: $2x - 3 > 3 - 4x$.

    a. $x > 1$
    b. $x < 1$
    c. $x > 2$
    d. $x < 2$

36. Solve for x: $\dfrac{24}{3x + 42} = \dfrac{2}{9}$

    a. 10
    b. 22
    c. 31
    d. 42

37. If $\dfrac{x}{y} = 5$ and $x = 25$, then what is the sum of x and y?

    a. 5
    b. 15
    c. 20
    d. 30

38. $(6x^3y^4z^2) \div (2xy^3z^5) =$

    a. $\dfrac{3x^2y}{z^3}$

    b. $\dfrac{x^2y}{3z^3}$

    c. $\dfrac{z^3}{3x^2y}$

    d. $3x^2yz^3$

39. Solve for x: $\dfrac{x^2 - 4x - 21}{x + 3} = 1$.
    a. 1
    b. 2
    c. 8
    d. 16

40. What is the solution set for the absolute value equation $|2x - 4| = 20$?
    a. $\{8, -12\}$
    b. $\{8, 12\}$
    c. $\{-8, 12\}$
    d. $\{-8, -12\}$

Science

45 Minutes

Read each question carefully and then select the correct answer. The correct answers will be found at the end of the test.

1. During plant cell replication, the division of the cytoplasm is called
   a. cytohydrolysis.
   b. cytokinesis.
   c. plasmolysis.
   d. cytoplasmosis.

2. Which of the following are classified as animals that eat only meat?
   a. Carnivores
   b. Herbivores
   c. Hecomposers
   d. Consumers

3. In which phase of mitosis do the chromosomes line up?
   a. Interphase
   b. Metaphase
   c. Prophase
   d. Anaphase

4. Digestive enzymes can be found in which cellular organelle?
   a. Lysosomes
   b. Mitochondria
   c. Golgi apparatus
   d. Ribosomes

5. The process by which an enzyme acts on the substrate can be described by the
   a. lock-and-key model.
   b. enzyme-and-substrate model.
   c. enzyme-folding model.
   d. catalytic model.

6. When an organism contains chloroplast in its cells, the color of the organism would most likely be
   a. orange.
   b. brown.
   c. yellow.
   d. green.

7. Refer to the following chart:

Object	Density in g/mL
W	0.56
X	1.45
Y	1.91
Z	8.45

Which object floats in water?
a. W
b. X
c. Y
d. Z

8. If 40 grams of a radioactive substance naturally decays to 10 grams after 16 days, what is the half-life of the substance?
a. 40 days
b. 8 days
c. 16 days
d. 10 days

9. A fertilized egg becomes a female fetus if the sperm contains which type of chromosome?
a. YY
b. XX
c. XY
d. X

10. In a food chain that contains producers, the original source of energy is most likely
a. the sun.
b. carbohydrates.
c. chlorophyll.
d. DNA.

11. Nitrogen bases, phosphate groups, and sugars containing five carbon atoms can be found in which of the following compounds?
a. Lipids
b. Proteins
c. Nucleic acids
d. Carbohydrates

12. Within the human body, which of the following distinguishes between threatening viruses and healthy tissue?
a. Leukocytes
b. Stem cells
c. Spleen
d. Bone marrow

13. Within the nose, which body part helps to filter the air being breathed?
    a. Epiglottis
    b. External meatus
    c. Cilia
    d. Tonsils

14. Of the following organisms, which is a vertebrate?
    a. Jellyfish
    b. Snake
    c. Spider
    d. Flatworm

15. Which of the following determines how high or low a sound is?
    a. Doppler effect
    b. Decibels
    c. Ultrasonic frequencies
    d. Pitch

16. Which chamber of the heart pumps oxygen-rich blood to the body?
    a. Left atrium
    b. Right atrium
    c. Left ventricle
    d. Right ventricle

17. An ionic compound made up of a metal and a nonmetal is called
    a. a salt.
    b. a base.
    c. an acid.
    d. a gel.

18. An atom with more protons in its nucleus has _____ an atom with fewer protons in its nucleus.
    a. a lesser nuclear charge than
    b. a greater nuclear charge than
    c. the same nuclear charge as
    d. no nuclear charge compared to

19. The half-life of a certain radioactive isotope is 5 days. How much of a 100-gram sample of this radioactive isotope will remain after 10 days?
    a. 25
    b. 50
    c. 75
    d. 100

20. What is the name of particle X in the following reaction?

$$^{232}_{90}\text{Th} \rightarrow {}^{228}_{88}\text{Ra} + X$$

    a. Deuterium
    b. Gamma radiation
    c. Beta particle
    d. Alpha particle

21. The electron configuration for neon is
    a. 2–5.
    b. 2–8.
    c. 2–18.
    d. 2–10.

22. The arrangement of the modern periodic table is based on atomic
    a. mass.
    b. number.
    c. radius.
    d. electronegativity.

23. Where on the periodic table are the nonmetals located?
    a. Upper right
    b. Upper left
    c. Lower right
    d. Lower left

24. Which two elements have chemical properties that are similar?
    a. H and He
    b. Fe and W
    c. Li and Be
    d. Mg and Ca

Element	# of Protons	# of Electrons	# of Neutrons
$^{18}_{8}\text{O}$	8		10
$^{14}_{6}\text{C}$		6	

25. How many protons are in $^{14}_{6}\text{C}$?
    a. 14
    b. 6
    c. 8
    d. 10

26. How many electrons are in $^{18}_{8}\text{O}$?
    a. 14
    b. 6
    c. 8
    d. 10

27. How many neutrons in $^{14}_{6}C$?
    a. 14
    b. 6
    c. 8
    d. 10

28. Which element has the lowest electronegativity?
    a. F
    b. Cl
    c. Br
    d. I

29. Which of the following elements has the greatest atomic radius?
    a. Strontium
    b. Fluorine
    c. Neon
    d. Cobalt

30. Which statement below is false?
    a. Hydrogen is a nonmetal.
    b. Aluminum is a semimetal.
    c. Calcium is a metal.
    d. Argon is a gas at room temperature.

31. Which compound contains a bond with no ionic character?
    a. CO
    b. CaO
    c. K_2O
    d. Na_2O

32. When K bonds with I, the
    a. electrons are shared.
    b. potassium gains electrons which are lost by iodine.
    c. two elements form a covalent compound.
    d. potassium loses one electron to iodine.

33. Which compound below has a nonpolar bond in which the electrons are being shared equally?
    a. H_2O
    b. NH_3
    c. Cl_2
    d. CH_4

34. In most living things, all of the following groups of chemicals can be found naturally *except*
    a. lipids.
    b. synthetic polymers.
    c. nucleic acids.
    d. carbohydrates.

35. Carbohydrates and starches must be changed to _____ so that they can be used by cells.
    a. glucose
    b. glycerin
    c. sucrose
    d. fructose

36. The process of food traveling throughout the digestive system is known as
    a. defecation.
    b. contractions.
    c. reverse peristalsis.
    d. peristalsis.

37. Accumulation of cholesterol leads to the hardening of the arteries. This is called
    a. vasoconstriction.
    b. venipuncture.
    c. atherosclerosis.
    d. hypertension.

38. The stomach and mouth are connected by the
    a. anus.
    b. esophagus.
    c. spinal column.
    d. epiglottis.

39. Which process named below includes the other three choices?
    a. Cellular respiration
    b. The Krebs cycle
    c. Anaerobic usage of glucose
    d. Electrons passing through the electron transport chain

40. Which color pairing of light is most beneficial for photosynthesis?
    a. Green/Yellow
    b. Green/Orange
    c. Green/Blue
    d. Red/Blue

41. The scientific nomenclature of an organism includes which of the following?
    a. Family and order
    b. Kingdom and phylum
    c. Genus and species
    d. Kingdom and class

42. Of the organisms below, which is classified as an herbivore?
    a. Snakes
    b. Birds
    c. Insects
    d. Green plants

43. In pea plants, shortness is recessive and tallness is dominant. If 50 percent of the F_2 generation of pea plants are short, then the F_1 generation could have been
    a. tt $\times$ tt.
    b. Tt $\times$ tt.
    c. TT $\times$ Tt.
    d. Tt $\times$ Tt.

44. Which process does the following equation represent?

    $$6CO_2 + \text{light energy} + 6H_2O \rightarrow C_6H_{12}O_6 + 6O_2$$

    a. Glycolysis
    b. Fermentation
    c. Photosynthesis
    d. Cellular respiration

45. Which of a plant's organs is responsible for sexual reproduction?
    a. Phloem
    b. Flower
    c. Bark
    d. Root

46. Which of the following processes is endothermic?
    a. Ice melting
    b. A piece of paper burning
    c. A bomb exploding
    d. An organism's metabolism producing a certain amount of heat

47. Which sentence best describes the following reaction?

    $$2H_2(g) + O_2(g) \rightarrow 2H_2O(l) + \text{heat}$$

    a. It is an endothermic reaction.
    b. It is an exothermic double replacement reaction.
    c. It is a synthesis reaction that is also exothermic.
    d. It is a decomposition that is also endothermic.

48. Which one of the following substances can be compressed the most?
    a. NaCl(aq)
    b. $Br_2(l)$
    c. $I_2(s)$
    d. $F_2(g)$

49. Definite shape and definite volume best describes a sample of
    a. $I_2(s)$.
    b. $Br_2(l)$.
    c. Cl(g).
    d. $F_2(g)$.

50. In which part of the heating curve below do water and ice exist at the same time?
    a. AB
    b. BC
    c. CD
    d. DE

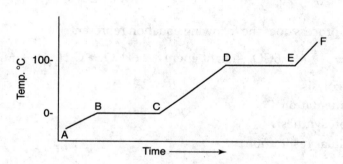

51. Which gas law below involves a variable not present in the other three?
    a. Boyle's Law
    b. Charles' Law
    c. Graham's Law
    d. Combined Gas Law

52. The smaller molecules that are responsible for the synthesis of starches are called
    a. lipids.
    b. monosaccharides.
    c. amino acids.
    d. nucleic acids.

53. Which of the following statements about catalysts is *false*?
    a. Catalysts speed up chemical reactions.
    b. Enzymes are catalysts.
    c. Catalysts are most effective at an optimum temperature and pH.
    d. Catalysts are destroyed while doing their job.

54. Chemical digestion does not occur in the
    a. mouth.
    b. small intestine.
    c. stomach.
    d. rectum.

55. What is the molar mass (the mass of one mole of a substance) of ammonia, NH_3?
    a. 10
    b. 17
    c. 8
    d. 15

56. What is the molar mass of calcium oxide, CaO?
    a. 56
    b. 28
    c. 640
    d. 320

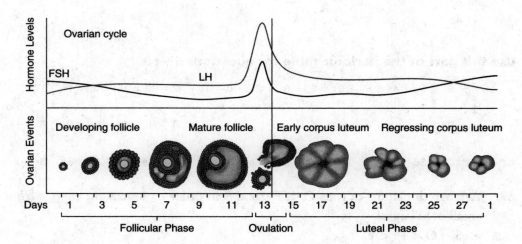

57. What correlation between FSH and LH can be drawn from the chart?
    a. Development of a follicle
    b. Follicle maturation
    c. Ovulation occurrence
    d. Prefertilized embryo

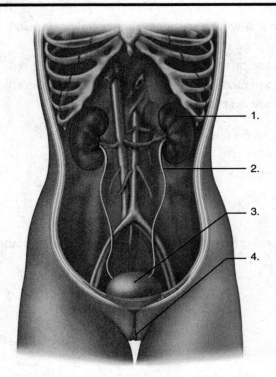

58. Which part of the urinary system stores urine?
    a. 1
    b. 2
    c. 3
    d. 4

Use this part of the periodic table for questions 59–60.

1	2	3	4	5	6	7	8	9	10	11	12	13	14	15	16	17	18
H																	He
Li	Be											B	C	N	O	F	Ne
Na	Mg											Al	Si	P	S	Cl	Ar
K	Ca	Sc	Ti	V	Cr	Mn	Fe	Co	Ni	Cu	Zn	Ga	Ge	As	Se	Br	Kr

59. Arrange the atoms or ions O, F, F^+, and S in order by ionization energy, from smallest to largest.
    a. $S < O < F^+ < F$
    b. $S < O < F < F^+$
    c. $F^+ < F < O < S$
    d. $O < F < F^+ < S$

60. Which of the following is a possible excited state for a Cl atom?
    a. $1s^2 2s^2 2p^6 3s^2 3p^4 3d^1$
    b. $1s^2 2s^2 2p^6 3s^2 3p^5$
    c. $1s^2 2s^2 2p^6 3s^2 3p^6$
    d. $1s^2 2s^2 2p^6 3s^2 3p^5 3d^1$

Practice Test 6

Verbal Ability

WORD KNOWLEDGE: Read each sentence carefully. Then, *on the basis of what is stated in the sentence*, select the correct answer to the incomplete statement.

1. The dressings for the bandages were alongside the sink. In other words, they were
    a. adjacent.
    b. obtuse.
    c. distracting.
    d. commendable.

2. The nurses in a ward got together to initiate their own successful protocol for allowing children to see their parents with the least amount of stress possible. They kept up this protocol because it was
    a. obsolete.
    b. ambitious.
    c. beneficial.
    d. probing.

3. After amassing an expensive baseball card collection, I was stunned by how soon it
    a. revered.
    b. depreciated.
    c. patronized.
    d. reconciled.

4. The hikers who were found after six days in the wilderness were
    a. disillusioned.
    b. ravenous.
    c. momentous.
    d. simultaneous.

5. The queen ruled an empire, yet she was subservient to the attacks of her cat. **Sub-servient** means
   a. amorphous.
   b. ignominious.
   c. docile.
   d. colloquial.

6. When a patient had a fever, in her delirium, she revealed personal secrets, but her nurse repeated none of what he heard because he was
   a. discreet.
   b. vindictive.
   c. scintillating.
   d. garish.

7. The politician's comments were so vitriolic that they only made the situation worse. **Vitriolic** means
   a. spurious.
   b. acerbic.
   c. superannuated.
   d. ebullient.

8. A person who wants to project an air of mystery wears a face that is
   a. translucent.
   b. fractious.
   c. inscrutable.
   d. risible.

9. People think presidents want their advisors to be obsequious. The truth is, better advice comes from someone who is
   a. degenerate.
   b. groveling.
   c. ignominious.
   d. emphatic.

10. Many people think it's pretentious to have wealthy kids show off their luxury car collection online. **Pretentious** means
    a. tenacious.
    b. ostentatious.
    c. pathological.
    d. nondescript.

11. Our guests left the house immaculate. Their manners were
    a. impeccable.
    b. boorish.
    c. infallible.
    d. materialistic.

12. The little toy poodle stood up to the German shepherd because she was
    a. congenial.
    b. pugnacious.
    c. illiterate.
    d. pacifying.

13. Even though Gilda was born on a farm, her travels made her quite cosmopolitan.
    Cosmopolitan means
    a. dispossessed.
    b. rampant.
    c. meandering.
    d. diverse.

14. The day that nurses are replaced by robots will be the triumph of
    a. gentility.
    b. dislocation.
    c. automation.
    d. bland.

15. My uncle could get 13 meals out of dozen eggs because he was very
    a. frugal.
    b. hybrid.
    c. contemptible.
    d. reputable.

16. After a night in the emergency room filled with tumult, it was nice to have a few
    hours of
    a. unification.
    b. chagrin.
    c. appropriation.
    d. serenity.

READING: There are five reading passages in this section. Read each passage carefully. Then on the basis of what you have read in the passage, select the best answer for each question.

PASSAGE 1

In the Civil War, the Battle of Shiloh in Tennessee is remembered as one of the bloodiest. Horrible hand-to-hand combat in a swamp resulted in 20,000 casualties. Both sides were equally affected. Each army had around 1,700 killed and 8,000 wounded. So many bodies covered the battlefield that the primitive medical staffs were overwhelmed. It took days to get to the injured. They lay in the mud as it rained and grew cold in a brisk April of 1862. The danger of infection, particularly gangrene, forced doctors of that day to amputate rather than disinfect. Yet the Shiloh killing fields became unique and what seemed to be a legend was born. As the soldiers lay in the mud puddles and muck moaning and waiting for a cruel death, their open wounds began to glow blue. As night came, witnesses reported seeing dots of greenish-blue light all over the area. The soldiers called it "angel's glow."

This phenomenon was well recorded because the doctors and nurses who eventually treated the wounded reported that a miracle had happened. Soldiers with the blue angel's glow were not dying. In fact, they were recovering much faster than others who didn't glow. They weren't becoming angels. They were instead becoming healthy. The angel's glow was some sort of gift of life. Soldiers were not that infected, but no one could explain why.

One hundred and fifty years later, in 2001, a high school student named Bill Martin came to Shiloh. He was a Civil War history buff, and when he heard the story of the mysterious angel glow, it sounded familiar. Bill's mother was a microbiologist at the USDA. She had told him about certain bacteria that were bioluminescent, which meant they could produce their own light. On his own, he and a friend did some research. For their school science fair, they presented their theory. They discovered that *Photorhabdus luminescens* is a bacteria that gives off a blue-green glow. It lives inside of nematodes, which are worms that are parasites. They invade the larvae of insects, where they vomit out the bacteria, which produces chemicals that kill the larvae and other microorganisms. Bill's theory was that the nematodes crawled into the open wounds and the "good" glowing bacteria killed off any "bad" bacteria that could cause infection. Yet there was one flaw in their theory: the "good" glowing type couldn't live inside the warmth of the human body.

It turns out that hypothermia saved these men's lives. The cold, damp swamp lowered their body temperatures, allowing the glowing bacteria to thrive. Once they got to the hospital, their bodies warmed up and killed off the glowing bacteria. Bill Martin solved the mystery, proving, as scientists have long known, that not all bacteria make us sick; some actually save lives.

17. The most important information this passage contains is about
    a. how bacteria can heal disease.
    b. a Civil War battle at Shiloh.
    c. explaining a phenomenon.
    d. a high school science fair.

18. Why was the blue light called angel's glow?
    a. It was assumed that sacred intervention was happening.
    b. It was the same blue light that angels give off in paintings.
    c. The dying soldiers were thought to be dying angels.
    d. The light was given off by angels in the open wounds.

19. Which is the best inference for how Bill Martin identified the bacteria?
    a. He looked at photographs from the Shiloh battlefield.
    b. He re-created the conditions that produced the bacteria.
    c. He was a trained microbiologist working for the government.
    d. He looked up all bioluminescent bacteria with blue light.

20. What allowed the bacteria to grow inside a human body?
    a. Nematodes
    b. Hypothermia
    c. Larvae
    d. Angel glow

21. The discovery of the beneficial effects of these bacteria would
    a. provide an answer to how these particular conditions worked.
    b. teach doctors how to save other future battlefield victims.
    c. help explain how other medical mysteries might be solved.
    d. lead to antibacterial medicines that would cure like a miracle.

22. We know the bacteria called angel's glow is not toxic to nematodes because
    a. it kills other microorganisms.
    b. it gives off a healing blue light.
    c. it dies off when temperatures rise.
    d. it exists inside their bodies.

PASSAGE 2

Do you have a headache? A sore throat? You can grab some kind of pill or syrup that will solve the problem. But be thankful you didn't live at other times in history when the cure for a headache was trepanation, which involved drilling or scraping a hole in your skull to let out the evil vapors. The Romans and Greeks regularly drained 30 percent to 40 percent of a sick person's blood supply to let out the "bad blood." They believed the body was filled with substances that had to be expelled. George Washington died this way. And it wasn't all that long ago that doctors prescribed the destruction of the brain's frontal lobes to cure mental illnesses, otherwise known as a lobotomy. Medical techniques have advanced exponentially in the past 100 years, but for centuries quack witch doctors and charlatans offered emergency room services that probably killed more people than they saved.

Even today, over 60 percent of the procedures performed in hospitals and home care have not been proven by any real study that has measured their effectiveness. They may well make people feel better and get well, but this has never been proven. In many ways, these cures are not all that different than the old folk remedy of lighting a candle in someone's ear to stop an earache, which some people still swear by. Today, treatments like oxygen therapy for acute myocardial infarction and bed rest for pregnancy have shown that they work, but there's no proof through a double-blind study to show why.

There must have been some result in ancient times that showed bleeding someone out was a good idea. Some poor patient must have felt better with a hole in her head, though it is hard to imagine why. Proper studies have shown that even the relatively modern technique from the late 1970s of exposing the bone marrow of breast cancer patients to radiation and then reimplanting it was ineffective and even fatal in some cases. So, why did oncologists prescribe it? Why did ancient doctors keep subjecting their patients to unproven treatments?

At the same time, many traditional ancient techniques, particularly plant medicines, have proven to be extremely effective. The fact that so many have been converted into pharmaceuticals verifies their worth. Even applying leeches to a sick person has been shown in studies to have some justifiable value. Double-blind studies have shown that leeches insert anticoagulants into the patient's blood, along with other helpful bioactive secretions.

At some point in the past there are lucky accidents or reckless practitioners who were willing to take the risk of a breakthrough. But whatever specialist or popular doctor of the day who gave mercury pills to the emperor of China in the 16th century must have been one confident caregiver. Qin Shi Huang wasn't a desperate cancer patient. He was the most powerful man in the world and was seeking the eternal life the strange, shiny liquid quicksilver seemed to have. Ultimately, raw liquid mercury actually killed the man who wanted to live forever.

23. One might infer from this passage that
    a. the author more or less approves of some ancient medical techniques.
    b. the author prefers modern medical techniques over ancient ones.
    c. medical practices should not be used if they haven't been proven.
    d. some patients are cured by having a hole drilled into their skull.

24. Which of the following statements is a conclusion reached by the author?
    a. Leech therapy like blood letting should not be used today.
    b. Trial and error has shown that some medical treatments work.
    c. Modern medicine needs to avoid ancient drugs and techniques.
    d. There is some proof that bad blood needs to be drained.

25. The major topic of this passage is
    a. doctors today could learn from ancient practitioners.
    b. many disproven medical ideas are still used today.
    c. medical treatments should be tested thoroughly.
    d. medicine is still using dangerous and barbaric techniques.

26. What was the extreme treatment for mental illness called?
    a. Oncology
    b. Trepanation
    c. Blood letting
    d. Lobotomy

27. How would the information in this article help nurses recommend treatments?
    a. It would help nurses demand a scientific study for any treatments they use.
    b. It would allow nurses to suggest other treatments doctors may not use.
    c. It would encourage nurses to study ancient techniques that are forgotten.
    d. It would encourage nurses to look for positive results from any treatment.

28. How did poor medical technique kill the Chinese emperor?
    a. He lost too much blood to bloodletting.
    b. He got an infection from trepanation.
    c. His bone marrow was exposed to radiation.
    d. He swallowed a poisonous substance.

PASSAGE 3

All that glitters is not aluminum metalized polyethylene terephthalate. It might even be mundane old Mylar. Everyone loves glitter, the sparkling pixie dust that creates magic at parties, discos, and Tinker Bell's touch, but it's actually just coated plastic bits. Humans love glitter as though it is some physical form of magic. However, the real reason we are so attracted to it has to do with our prehistoric ancestors searching for water. In glitter, subliminally we see that distant dancing glint of sunlight reflecting off the surface of water, the substance that keeps us alive.

No doubt the glimmer and refraction of diamonds in sunlight or the starburst twinkle of polished silver are integral to our fascination with glitter, yet little is known about the manufacture and application of the miniature prisms spread all over Christmas ornaments, disco balls, and even our lips. Surprisingly, only two factories in New Jersey make the bulk of it. And they refuse to say who buys their product and how it is used in its many forms. Why this is a secret has everything to do with the allure of the sparkles, and that companies don't want you to know they are using it to draw you in like the reflection of a stream calling out to our early ancestors.

Today's glitter starts out as clear sheets of plastic of the same sort used in water bottles, so it's FDA approved. In the past, ground glass and crushed mica stone were the first forms of glitter. Early German Christmas ornaments and decorations had the twinkle of moonlight on objects below from chips of mica that imitated crystalline snowflakes. But the invention of Mylar created glitter for the masses, as this thin, durable clear plastic can be chopped into the tiniest pieces, which are then coated with aluminum through a secret evaporation process that takes place in a vacuum to create a substrate across both sides of the polymer pieces. The colors of glitter from startling pinks to haunting purples are engineered to tease the eye. Rainbow-causing glitter has holographic patterns etched on it. Each layer is so thin that it's half the wavelength of light, or about 230 nanometers. A human hair is about 100,000 nanometers thick.

The problem is that glitter isn't going anywhere. It is so fine that it's ubiquitous. And it's nonbiodegradable, which is why President Obama signed a bill in 2015 to keep it out of makeup meant to be washed off. With our current fear of eating or drinking microplastics like glitter bits, a push for cellulose-based glitter is gaining. Glitter is everywhere, from football helmets to animal feces (easy to find with a flashlight after tracking scientists glitterize their food). It's in toothpaste and explosives, and it dusts crime scenes as well as top secret rockets. Its microbeads litter cosmetics. The only way humans are going to avoid glitter is breaking our addiction to it, but then we'd have to be no longer fascinated by the shiny shimmer of sunlight off water.

29. Which of the following titles is best for this passage?
    a. "How Glitter Is Made"
    b. "Glitter's Threat to the Environment"
    c. "The Deep Allure of Glitter"
    d. "All That Glitters Is Not Gold"

30. According to the passage, the sparkles of glitter come from
    a. aluminum.
    b. Mylar.
    c. mica.
    d. water.

31. Why did the government ban glitter in wash-off cosmetics?
    a. Because it is hard to clean up
    b. Because the pieces were too small
    c. To keep it out of the water supply
    d. To keep it from being FDA approved

32. After reading this article, one could conclude that
    a. more companies will get into the business of making glitter.
    b. glitter made from cellulose will be just as popular as plastic glitter.
    c. human beings will never be able to resist their love of glitter.
    d. companies using glitter fear consumers will avoid their products.

33. What produces the rainbow effect in some glitter?
    a. pixie dust
    b. holograms
    c. tiny prisms
    d. polyethylene terephthalate

34. It can be inferred from the passage that
    a. someday glitter will be added to almost every product.
    b. the reflective light off glitter is related to a basic need.
    c. modern glitter will never fully replace ground glass and mica.
    d. the thickness of the substrate should be 100,000 nanometers.

PASSAGE 4

One of the greatest success stories of vaccines and public health is the happy saga of the scourge of polio. The poliovirus, known as poliomyelitis, is highly infectious, but only in relatively recent history did it become a paralyzer and killer. A painting on an Egyptian stele (a decorated stone often used in tombs) shows a young man with a withered leg steadying himself with a cane. This is proof that the disease existed 3,500 years ago, long before it became widespread. In 1789, an English physician, Michael Underwood, identified four cases of the disease. At this point it was a rare localized disease, but by the turn of the 20th century, it suddenly became a widespread endemic disease that threatened the entire world.

Industrialization brought larger populations to the cities, and in 1916 the first large epidemic of polio struck the United States in New York, where 9,000 cases occurred, resulting in 2,300 deaths. In 1921, the future president Franklin Delano Roosevelt became infected at the relatively old age of 39, and although he disguised many of his symptoms so that voters would continue to elect him, he put a public face on a horrible disease. The virus's damage to the spinal cord caused painful contractions and the loss of the ability to walk, which struck fear through the population. Chest paralysis forced the development of iron lungs, artificial breathing apparatuses that aided respiration and kept thousands alive. Many children suffered eye paralysis. By the early 1950s, polio outbreaks resulted in more than 15,000 new cases per year.

The first attempts at developing a vaccine were horrible failures, resulting in many deaths. Then science triumphed in 1952, when Dr. Jonas Salk developed the first successful vaccine. Newspaper headlines trumpeted him as the savior of children, and church bells rang out. Dr. Albert Sabin pioneered the first oral vaccine, allowing easy widespread prevention. Within five years, polio cases dropped 90 percent. The Global Polio Eradication Initiative inoculated more than 2.5 billion children and eradicated the disease from most countries. The last 1 percent resisted due to political strife and the ability of the disease to still spread from a single case. Within a few decades, the scourge that affected millions had been all but wiped off the face of the Earth.

35. The best title for this passage is
    a. "The Impossibility of Curing Polio."
    b. "A President Fights a Deadly Disease."
    c. "The Scourge of Polio before the Cure."
    d. "It Takes the World to Stop a Worldwide Epidemic."

36. The most important breakthrough in combating polio is
    a. developing a vaccine.
    b. isolating potential victims.
    c. the creation of iron lungs.
    d. a president getting the disease.

37. Polio's ability to spread easily from a single case means that
    a. vaccines have only limited effect on it.
    b. it was very difficult to identify and isolate.
    c. ancient peoples were equally affected by it.
    d. it has to be eradicated nearly 100 percent to stop it.

38. How does the story of eradicating polio apply to unknown diseases in the future?
    a. It means that all diseases can some day disappear.
    b. It suggests current research is the key.
    c. It shows the power of vaccinations.
    d. It offers hope that epidemics are a thing of the past.

39. The author is suggesting that
    a. most viral diseases can be eradicated.
    b. a concerted worldwide effort was needed.
    c. the oral vaccination should have been developed first.
    d. doctors should not have attempted the first fatal vaccines.

40. Why were people so terrified by the polio virus if it has been around for 3,500 years?
    a. Ancient Egyptians had the disease, but it had not posed a threat until recently.
    b. Increased populations of cities caused the virus to spread into an epidemic.
    c. When the president became ill with the disease, people began to get scared.
    d. In the 1800s, the disease showed it could lead to epidemics no one could stop.

PASSAGE 5

Spiders, the most prolific predators in the world, feed upon countless billions of insects, and without them, humans would have been overrun with mosquitoes, butterflies, and gnats long ago. Spiders spin sophisticated, complexly designed webs whose engineering assures them success; they produce silk that is five times stronger than steel and can stretch to four times its length; they can live underwater, produce neurotoxins to paralyze their prey, and dissolve their victims into liquid so they can drink them in. Yet recent studies have proven that spiders have another super power: they can fly.

Scientists have suspected that arachnids move from place to place at times by hitching a ride on the wind with a technique called ballooning, because the spider shoots out a strand of its silk and appears to hang on to it as the prevailing winds carry it aloft with air currents. However, this behavior has been misunderstood, and although some spiders balloon with the wind, they do so only in light circulation. Instead, scientists suspected that something intricate was at play. Then an astrophysicist at the University of Hawaii named Peter Gorham unearthed an account from 1832 by the naturalist Charles Darwin, who witnessed millions of miniature spiders blanketing his ship 60 miles offshore of Argentina. Gorham did the calculations and proved that in a chalkboard formula at least, spiders could be hitchhiking on electrical currents, which actually was first proposed as a possibility in the 1800s.

Earth has a negative charge, and the upper atmosphere, the positively charged ionosphere, is fully positive from 50 to 600 miles, which considerably extends the spider's range of flight.

It took biologists Erica Morley and Daniel Robert to prove how spiders accomplish this evolutionary marvel. The scientists built a control box with an artificial electrical field and employed lasers to discover that miniature hairs on the spiders' feet called trichobothria can sense electrical fields. Spider silk picks up a negative charge from the air, and then spiders perform a little dance called tiptoeing, jacking their abdomens into the air until they lift off—even when there is no air movement in the box. To confirm their theory, the biologists then disconnected the artificial current in the box and the spiders plummeted out of the sky.

Complicated and interrelated motivations are suggested by this behavior, as scientists now can speculate that spiders could use ballooning to escape ecosystems that cannot support sufficient insect populations they need as food, and the technique could also be used to colonize every inch of the Earth, as well as to flee from predators effortlessly. The technical term for this ability is electrostatic repulsion. Bees, sharks, and cockroaches also decipher electrical fields—unlike humans—so it is theoretically possible that other organisms have this evolutionary advantage over us, unless we learn how spiders know when to ride the electric grid. With that knowledge, we might be able to keep spiders from leaving an ecosystem, which could collapse without its apex insect predator, or we might be able to control rogue insect populations like fruit flies overwhelming orchards at harvest time, and perhaps, wildly, humans will ascertain somehow to ride polar electricity themselves.

41. Which of these topics is the main focus of this passage?
    a. Electrical currents in the air
    b. Amazing facts about spiders
    c. Darwin's theories about spiders
    d. Discoveries about spider ballooning

42. What causes spiders to fly long distances?
    a. Interaction between positive and negative charges
    b. The wind getting ahold of a strand of their silk
    c. The need to pursue distant populations of insects
    d. Swinging from place to place with strong silk strands

43. Which fact disproved the notion that spiders ride the wind?
    a. It is not mathematically possible for them to fly.
    b. They only fly when there is little air circulation.
    c. They have been discovered too high in the air where there isn't wind.
    d. Their web silk is not strong enough to support their weight.

44. Which part of a spider can sense electrical signals?
    a. Its web
    b. Neurotoxins
    c. Trichobothria
    d. Electrostatic repulsion

45. One might infer from this passage that
    a. many organisms have powers we don't realize.
    b. spiders can travel farther and faster in a thunderstorm.
    c. cockroaches can also fly using electrical currents.
    d. the biologists proved spiders can't fly without wind.

46. How would the facts of this passage help scientists to understand other animal behavior?
    a. A proper mathematical formula is necessary to explain animal behavior.
    b. Electricity in the atmosphere probably controls a wide variety of animals.
    c. A carefully controlled experiment can verify what is observed in nature.
    d. Other insects will probably develop the ability to fly to escape spiders.

47. The surgeon was so immersed in his work that he didn't even hear the fire bell. **Immersed** means
    a. distracted.
    b. repulsed.
    c. agitated.
    d. absorbed.

48. After rising gang violence, some families moved out seeking
    a. camouflage.
    b. sanctuary.
    c. engagement.
    d. conviction.

49. A medicine whose purpose is to exterminate a condition will act to have it
    a. eradicated.
    b. diminished.
    c. enlightened.
    d. transformed.

50. A child on a playground who is unruly is
    a. sophisticated.
    b. extraordinary.
    c. wayward.
    d. competent.

51. The hurricane caused a devastating public health crisis, but the failure of the water sanitation system proved to be
    a. legitimate.
    b. renowned.
    c. phenomenal.
    d. disastrous.

52. The review board is likely to exonerate the nurses involved in the incident, but the doctors could be held responsible. **Exonerate** means
    a. recant.
    b. execrate.
    c. mollify.
    d. vindicate.

53. The speaker's comments were so filled with criticism that it sounded more like
    a. an elegy.
    b. a martinet.
    c. a diatribe.
    d. a montage.

54. In the operating room, nurses, surgeons, and specialists have to perform together as a team. They have to be a unit whose work must be
    a. cohesive.
    b. irreparable.
    c. fecund.
    d. pusillanimous.

55. In an average day, nurses face a myriad of problems, and the trick is not to be overwhelmed. **Myriad** means
    a. multitude.
    b. deficiency.
    c. affectation.
    d. faction.

56. Although he had an ordered mind, his personal habits were
    a. stereotypical.
    b. redundant.
    c. negligible.
    d. slovenly.

57. When the children came into the room boisterous and covered with snow after sledding, it felt like the storm outside had come inside. **Boisterous** means
    a. emancipated.
    b. fraught.
    c. energetic.
    d. glib.

58. Despite the chaos of the emergency room, the nurses there were calm and peaceful. Their manner was
    a. devout.
    b. serene.
    c. disapproving.
    d. intolerable.

59. The reviewer described a sublime dining experience at the new restaurant because the food was
    a. exquisite.
    b. obscure.
    c. mediocre.
    d. profound.

60. After the X-ray equipment broke down, the experts found that although the fired technician's work was unprofessional, his intentions were not
    a. titanic.
    b. waning.
    c. authentic.
    d. malicious.

Mathematics

Work each problem carefully. Use scrap paper to do your calculations.

1. The average cost of a stay in a hospital is about $3,900. It is projected to rise by 18 percent over the next decade. What would a patient be paying for an average hospital stay in 10 years?
   a. $4,200
   b. $4,602
   c. $4,815
   d. $5,700

2. $-36 \div -6 =$
   a. -42
   b. 42
   c. -6
   d. 6

3. In one minute, a patient's pulse rate is recorded as 90. In 20 seconds, what would the recorded pulse rate be?
   a. 20
   b. 30
   c. 40
   d. 60

4. $\sqrt{63} =$
   a. $3\sqrt{7}$
   b. $2 \times 30 + 3$
   c. $9\sqrt{54}$
   d. 9×7

5. $\dfrac{x^2 - xy}{y^2 - xy} =$
   a. $-\dfrac{x}{y}$
   b. $\dfrac{x}{y}$
   c. $\dfrac{x^3 y}{y^3 x}$
   d. $\dfrac{x^2}{y^2}$

6. In order to give a patient 800,000 units of a penicillin solution, how many milliliters from a 2-milliliter syringe containing 1,200,000 units in aqueous solution should be injected?

    a. $\dfrac{1}{4}$

    b. $\dfrac{2}{3}$

    c. $\dfrac{3}{4}$

    d. $1\dfrac{1}{4}$

7. 96 is 80% of what number?

    a. 120
    b. 124
    c. 80
    d. 100

8. At 1 p.m., an elderly patient's temperature was 101.7°F. For half a day, her temperature rose. The average rise was 0.25°F every hour. What was the patient's temperature at 1 a.m.?

    a. 100.2°
    b. 102.2°
    c. 103.2°
    d. 104.7°

9. Simplify: $8 - 4(a - 5b)$

    a. $8 - 4a + 20b$
    b. $8a + 20b$
    c. $4a - 5b$
    d. $8 - 4a - 20b$

10. 2/3 (½ + ⅛) =

    a. $\dfrac{3}{16}$

    b. $\dfrac{1}{8}$

    c. $\dfrac{6}{12}$

    d. $\dfrac{5}{12}$

11. How many milliliters are in 2.74 liters?

    a. 0.274
    b. 2.74
    c. 27.40
    d. 2,740

12. What is the volume of a box with sides of 12 cubic m, 18 cubic m, and 10 cubic m?
    a. 120 m
    b. 1,180 cubic m
    c. 216 cubic m
    d. 2,160 cubic m

13. $\sqrt{72} + \sqrt{108} =$
    a. $\sqrt{90}$
    b. $3\sqrt{2}$
    c. $9\sqrt{2}$
    d. $18\sqrt{2}$

14. If a patient's output of fluids was 400 milliliters, how much would this represent in liters?
    a. $\dfrac{1}{10}$
    b. $\dfrac{1}{3}$
    c. $\dfrac{5}{6}$
    d. $\dfrac{2}{5}$

15. In one year at a nursing school, 12.5 percent of the incoming students came from out of state. Which fraction best represents the proportion of students coming in from out of state to study there?
    a. $\dfrac{1}{12}$
    b. $\dfrac{1}{10}$
    c. $\dfrac{1}{8}$
    d. $\dfrac{1}{6}$

16. A patient took 3 pills of a drug whose dosage was 625 mg each. The guidelines warn that no more than 1.5 grams of the drug should be taken safely. How much did the patient overdose or underdose in grams?
    a. Overdose by 0.375 gm
    b. Overdose by 6.25 gm
    c. Underdose by 3.75 gm
    d. Underdose by 1.875 gm

17. A hospital room entrance forms a triangle with a 3-m base and a 6-m height. What area would this triangle have?
    a. 5 m
    b. 7 m
    c. 9 m
    d. 18 m

18. If $7a = 4b + 11$, and $a = 5$, then $b =$
    a. 3.
    b. 5.
    c. 6.
    d. 8.

19. How many grams are in 345 mg if one gram contains 1,000 milligrams?
    a. 3.45
    b. 34.5
    c. 0.345
    d. 0.0345

20. The number 175 is what percentage of 265?
    a 48 percent
    b. 125 percent
    c. 60 percent
    d. 66 percent

21. $593.1 - 36.821 =$
    a. 224.89
    b. 629.921
    c. 556.28
    d. 556.279

22. During an annual blood drive, volunteers donated 7 ¼ quarts of blood. A multiple car collision needed 3 ¼ pints of blood that same day. What is the amount of blood donated that day after the pints needed for the accident are used?
    a 11 ¼ pints
    b. 2 quarts
    c. 11 ¾ pints
    d. 7 pints

23. Latoya and Carmen have together earned 82 credits during their schooling. Latoya has 7 more credits than Carmen. Which of these equations shows their total amount of credits, if x represents the credits Carmen has?
    a. $82 - x = 7$
    b. $x + 7x = 82$
    c. $2x + 7 = 82$
    d. $x + 7 = 82$

24. When counting from 74 to 82, which prime number would you encounter?
    a. 74
    b. 77
    c. 79
    d. 81

25. Study these similar triangles. Note that all sides are corresponding. What is the length of x?

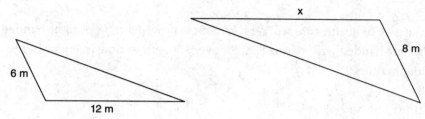

    a. 10 m
    b. 12 m
    c. 14 m
    d. 16 m

26. $5z^3 \times 4z^5 =$
    a. $1z^{15}$
    b. $2z^{15}$
    c. $20z^8$
    d. $1z^2$

27. What is the approximate ratio of men to women in nursing if there are 330,000 male registered nurses and 3,200,000 female registered nurses today?
    a. 1:10
    b. 1:12
    c. 1:32
    d. 2:25

28. Which of the following percentages equals 0.41?
    a. 0.041 percent
    b. 0.41 percent
    c. 4.1 percent
    d. 41 percent

29. $\dfrac{5}{6} \div \dfrac{2}{3} =$
    a. $\dfrac{5}{9}$
    b. $\dfrac{2}{3}$
    c. $1\dfrac{1}{4}$
    d. $2\dfrac{1}{4}$

30. Study these fractions. Choose the one that represents the smallest amount.

    a. $\dfrac{1}{8-4}$

    b. $\dfrac{1}{8\times4}$

    c. $\dfrac{1}{8\div4}$

    d. $\dfrac{1}{8+4}$

31. In a survey of health care workers, statistics showed a ratio of right-handed writers to left-handed writers was 8:2. For every 50 lefties, how many would be right-handed writers?

    a. 8
    b. 100
    c. 200
    d. 400

32. While counting a patient's contractions over 5 minutes, results of 6, 10, 16, 5, and 3 were recorded. What is the average number of contractions over that time period?

    a. 8
    b. 12
    c. 10
    d. 9

33. A liquid medicine given to elderly patients who have difficulty swallowing provides 25 mg of medication for every 10-ml dose. In order to provide 85 mg of this medication, how many milliliters would have to be dispensed?

    a. 10
    b. 30
    c. 34
    d. 165

34. What is 29 percent of 486?

    a. 97.2
    b. 120.8
    c. 140.94
    d. 14,094

35. Hospital policy states that if 3/4 of the patients in the ICU are on oxygen, the staff needs to requisition additional tanks to avoid any shortages. At the start of the shift, 10 patients were on oxygen and the ICU was using 24 beds. How many more patients would have to be on oxygen before additional tanks needed to be requisitioned?
    a. 3
    b. 4
    c. 15
    d. 8

36. $86.36 \div 0.34 =$
    a. 254
    b. 25.4
    c. 2.54
    d. 2.054

37. $-22 + 19 =$
    a. 3
    b. −3
    c. −41
    d. 41

38. $7,345 - 957 =$
    a. 6,382
    b. 7,388
    c. 6,388
    d. 6,358

39. How would you round off the number 9,452.0872 to the nearest hundredth?
    a. 9,452
    b. 9,452.1
    c. 9,453.11
    d. 9,452.09

40. Which one of the following mathematical statements is true?
    a. $0.3 = \dfrac{3}{100}$
    b. $0.048 = \dfrac{48}{100}$
    c. $0.0294 = \dfrac{294}{10,000}$
    d. $0.116 = \dfrac{11}{6}$

Science

Read each question carefully, and then select the correct answer.

1. If your parents both have a combination of dominant and recessive alleles for a characteristic, you would not display or show that trait if your alleles were
   a. AA.
   b. Aa.
   c. aA.
   d. aa.

2. What structural organization level of the body does the stomach represent?
   a. Cellular level
   b. Tissue level
   c. Organ level
   d. System level

3. An example of a long bone is the
   a. sternum.
   b. patella.
   c. vertebra.
   d. humerus.

4. An example of a polar covalent bond would be
   a. $\ddot{\text{Cl}} :: \ddot{\text{Cl}}$
   b. $\text{H} : \text{H}$
   c. $\text{H} : \ddot{\text{Cl}} :$
   d. $\text{H} : \overset{\text{H}}{\underset{\text{H}}{\text{C}}} : \text{H}$

5. The term *hyperventilation* refers to
   a. a solution that causes cells to shrink through osmosis.
   b. elevated body temperature.
   c. movement beyond the normal range.
   d. a rate of inhalation and exhalation higher than necessary.

6. Scientists tested bacteria in a laboratory by exposing them to a weak dose of penicillin, and then exposed whatever offspring that survived to increasingly stronger doses of penicillin. They also developed individual bacteria that had never been

exposed to penicillin, and then exposed them to penicillin. What were the scientists trying to prove about evolution?

a. Only bacteria that were exposed to penicillin developed resistance.

b. Penicillin did not work on bacteria that had never been exposed to it.

c. Resistance to penicillin was not the result of simple survival.

d. Penicillin evolved over generations until it no longer killed bacteria.

7. The part of a plant's reproductive system that is analogous to the human male's testes is the

a. anther.

b. petal.

c. stigma.

d. ovule.

8. In plants, a seed would develop after it is fertilized in the

a. stigma.

b. sepal.

c. peduncle.

d. ovary.

9. The acceleration a skydiver achieves before he pulls the parachute is

a. 32 feet per second.

b. terminal velocity.

c. gravitational attraction.

d. 50 miles an hour.

Use the following information to answer questions 10 and 11.

If your BMI is less than 18.5, it falls within the underweight range.

If your BMI is 18.5 to 24.9, it falls within the normal or healthy weight range.

If your BMI is 25.0 to 29.9, it falls within the overweight range.

If your BMI is 30.0 or higher, it falls within the obese range.

BMI	19	20	21	22	23	24	25	26	27	28	29	30	31	32	33	34	35
Height (inches)	Body Weight (pounds)																
58	91	96	100	105	110	115	119	124	129	134	138	143	148	153	158	162	167
59	94	99	104	109	114	119	124	128	133	138	143	148	153	158	163	168	173
60	97	102	107	112	118	123	128	133	138	143	148	153	158	163	168	174	179
61	100	106	111	116	122	127	132	137	143	148	153	158	164	169	174	180	185
62	104	109	115	120	126	131	136	142	147	153	158	164	169	175	180	186	191
63	107	113	118	124	130	135	141	146	152	158	163	169	175	180	186	191	197
64	110	116	122	128	134	140	145	151	157	163	169	174	180	186	192	197	204
65	114	120	126	132	138	144	150	156	162	168	174	180	186	192	198	204	210
66	118	124	130	136	142	148	155	161	167	173	179	186	192	198	204	210	216
67	121	127	134	140	146	153	159	166	172	178	185	191	198	204	211	217	223
68	125	131	138	144	151	158	164	171	177	184	190	197	203	210	216	223	230
69	128	135	142	149	155	162	169	176	182	189	196	203	209	216	223	230	236
70	132	139	146	153	160	167	174	181	188	195	202	209	216	222	229	236	243
71	136	143	150	157	165	172	179	186	193	200	208	215	222	229	236	243	250
72	140	147	154	162	169	177	184	191	199	206	213	221	228	235	242	250	258
73	144	151	159	166	174	182	189	197	204	212	219	227	235	242	250	257	265
74	148	155	163	171	179	186	194	202	210	218	225	233	241	249	256	264	272
75	152	160	168	176	184	192	200	208	216	224	232	240	248	256	264	272	279
76	156	164	172	180	189	197	205	213	221	230	238	246	254	263	271	279	287

10. A person 5 feet 8 inches tall who weighs 153 pounds would have a BMI of _____ and be considered _____.
    a. 20, underweight
    b. 23, healthy
    c. 26, overweight
    d. 31, obese

11. Someone with a BMI index of 33 and a height of 76 inches who wants to diet until he is in the normal or healthy weight range would have to lose approximately
    a. 15 lbs.
    b. 25 lbs.
    c. 66 lbs.
    d. 85 lbs.

12. A car traveling at 25 miles an hour hits a tree and is badly damaged. The same car after it is repaired hits another tree, but this time it is totaled. Its speed was 50 miles an hour the second time. How much greater was the kinetic energy of the repaired car than the original car?
    a. The same
    b. Doubled
    c. Tripled
    d. Quadrupled

13. If a taxonomist discovers a living organism from outer space and wants to begin classifying it by its similarities with living things on Earth, the first consideration she should make is its
    a. kingdom.
    b. phylum.
    c. domain.
    d. family.

14. Which of the following are parasites?
    a. Microorganisms living inside cows
    b. Remoras attached to sharks
    c. Cows eating grass
    d. Tapeworms in the intestines

15. What distinguishes a tincture from an emulsion?
    a. A tincture needs an emulsifier, and an emulsion needs a tincture.
    b. A tincture is a heterogeneous mixture, and an emulsion is homogeneous.
    c. A tincture has alcohol as a solvent, and an emulsion is liquid dispersed in liquid.
    d. A tincture is a solvent, and an emulsion is a solute.

16. Which part of the brain regulates heartbeat, breathing, and blood vessel diameter?
    a. Cerebrum
    b. Medulla oblongata
    c. Cerebellum
    d. Midbrain

17. Which of the following conducts motor nerve impulses from the brain to the rest of the body?
    a. Thalamus
    b. Cerebellum
    c. Pons
    d. Spinal cord

Use the following graph of a chemical reaction to answer questions 18 and 19.

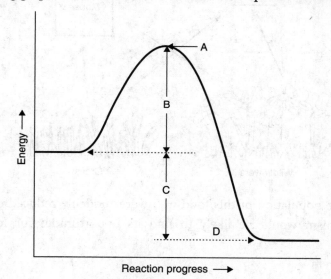

18. Which areas described in the line graph by letters would show the activated complex?
    a. A
    b. B
    c. C
    d. D

19. If a catalyst were to be introduced to the reaction shown on the line graph, what would change the most?
    a. Progress of activated complex
    b. Activation energy
    c. Energy released by reaction
    d. Energy of products

Use the food web diagram shown below to answer questions 20, 21, and 22.

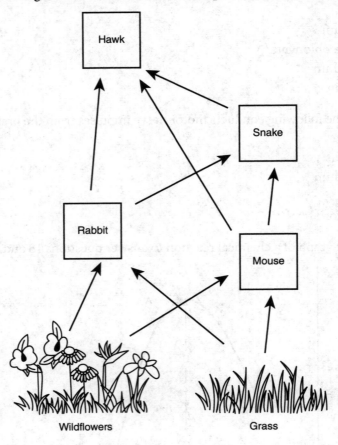

20. If the mouse population of this food web were suddenly reduced dramatically, which organism would be likely to find its opportunities for food sources diminish?
    a. Wildflowers
    b. Rabbit
    c. Snake
    d. Hawk

21. Which of these food chains shows the correct flow of energy in this food web?
    a. Hawk –> rabbit –> mouse –> grass
    b. Wildflowers –> mouse –> snake –> hawk
    c. Grass –> snake –> hawk –> rabbit
    d. Wildflowers –> grass –> rabbit –> snake –> hawk

22. If another member of the food chain were added to this diagram, what would its arrows point to or what arrows would point to it?
    a. Every organism would point to *decomposer*.
    b. Sunlight would be added as a *producer* pointing to every organism.
    c. Wolves would be added as a *primary consumer* of snakes and point to it.
    d. Frogs would be added as a *secondary consumer* of grass, which would point it.

23. How would you write the formula for sucrose?
    a. $C_{12}H_{22}O_{11}$
    b. CH_3COOH
    c. $NaHCO_3$
    d. NaCIO

24. Liquid drain cleaner is a strong base. What is its likely pH?
    a. 0
    b. 2
    c. 7
    d. 14

25. In the periodic table, elements in a column have similar
    a. atomic numbers.
    b. principal energy levels.
    c. chemical properties.
    d. atomic mass.

26. Which information in a periodic table would tell you that the noble gases are inert?
    a. Atomic number
    b. Number of valence electrons
    c. Element symbol
    d. Average atomic mass

27. The organ that secretes bile and processes drugs is the
    a. pancreas.
    b. liver.
    c. gallbladder.
    d. colon.

28. After broken-down food leaves the stomach, it passes into the
    a. appendix.
    b. ascending colon.
    c. duodenum.
    d. liver.

29. If you were referring to an injury in the hand as well as the shoulder on the same side of the body, which directional term would describe the position of the hand injury to the shoulder wound?
    a. Distal
    b. Proximal
    c. Inferior
    d. Posterior

30. After playing basketball, a woman experienced swelling many hours after she played. The swelling was caused by
    a. bleeding from blood vessels at areas of injury.
    b. torn muscles that support the knee.
    c. dislocation of the tibia relative to the femur.
    d. overproduction of synovial fluid.

Use the information in the following graph to answer questions 31 and 32.

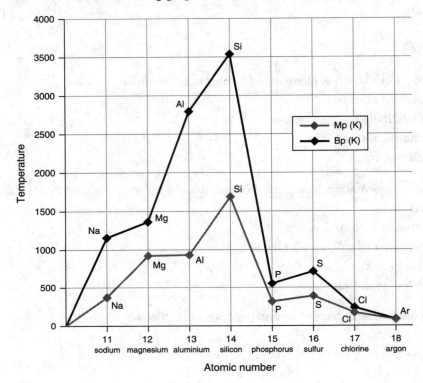

31. Which of these elements has the greatest difference between their melting and boiling points?
    a. Sodium
    b. Aluminum
    c. Silicon
    d. Argon

32. These are all Period 2 elements. Why are the properties of their boiling and melting points so different?
    a. Not all Period 2 elements have similar properties.
    b. Their atomic numbers vary greatly.
    c. Some metals absorb energy to retain their forms.
    d. Their atomic structures are different.

33. Which of these properties are found only in base solutions?
    a. They cause some chemical dyes to change color.
    b. They taste bitter and feel slippery to the touch.
    c. They react with certain metals to produce hydrogen gas.
    d. They form water and salt after reacting with compounds.

34. Which of the following mathematical expressions states Boyle's law of gases?
    a. $\dfrac{V_1}{T_1} = \dfrac{V_2}{T_2}$

    b. $\dfrac{P_1 \cdot V_1}{T_1} = \dfrac{P_2 \cdot V_2}{T_2}$

    c. $\dfrac{P_1}{T_1} = \dfrac{P_2}{T_2}$

    d. $P_1 \cdot V_1 = P_2 \cdot V_2$

35. A patient was standing too close to an extremely loud explosion. Many parts of his ear were damaged by the blast. He is particularly bothered by constant dizziness. Which part of his ear was damaged to cause him vertigo?
    a. Outer ear
    b. Tympanic membrane
    c. Vestibular apparatus
    d. Cochlea

36. Before running a marathon, runners eat foods that will provide extra energy late in the race. Otherwise, runners would hit "the wall" as their muscles deplete stored energy. Which organic compound do they eat?
    a. Lipids
    b. Cellulose
    c. Monosaccharides
    d. Amino acids

37. Trees will not grow in the terrestrial biome known as
    a. deserts.
    b. tundra.
    c. taiga.
    d. savanna.

38. The most useful type of microscope for viewing extremely small objects is
    a. pocket.
    b. compound.
    c. digital.
    d. electron.

39. A car's speed as demonstrated by this graph is

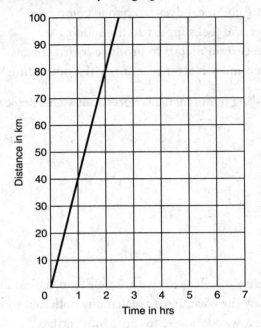

a. 22 km/hr.
b. 38 km/hr.
c. 40 km/hr.
d. 50 km/hr.

40. The Celsius scale is easier to use than the Fahrenheit scale because
a. everyone knows that normal human body temperature is 98.6°.
b. because to convert to Celsius you have to use a complicated formula.
c. it has more gradients in the temperatures most people use daily.
d. the freezing point and boiling point of water are easy multiples of 10.

Use the following diagram of ocean waves to answers questions 41 and 42.

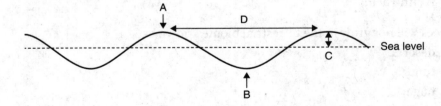

41. The amplitude of these waves is described by
a. A.
b. B.
c. C.
d. D.

42. The frequency of the ocean waves shown would be
    a. the speed of the wave through different mediums.
    b. 3 hertz.
    c. equal to the energy shown between the crest and trough.
    d. the number of crests passing A in a certain time.

43. A good source of fiber in your diet would come from eating
    a. fish.
    b. blueberries.
    c. apples.
    d. sweet potatoes.

Use the food diagram and food pyramid below to answer questions 44 and 45.

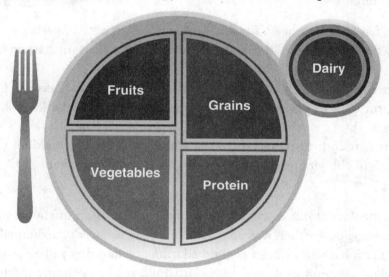

ChooseMyPlate.gov

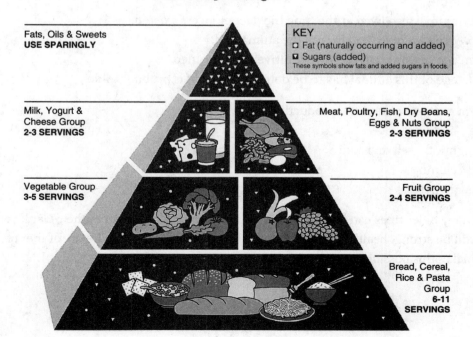

44. Compare these two food diagrams for healthy eating. What is the biggest difference between recommended service size in the new plate versus the older pyramid?
    a. The pyramid suggests more grains than the plate does.
    b. The pyramid suggests more vegetables than fruits than the plate does.
    c. Unlike the pyramid, the plate has equal amounts of proteins and diary.
    d. Unlike the pyramid, the plate fails to offer guidance for amounts or servings.

45. The type of food not shown in one diagram but shown in the other is
    a. dairy.
    b. fruits.
    c. oils, fats, sweets.
    d. pasta, nuts.

46. A victim has suffered a heart attack as well as a broken neck or perhaps a broken back in a building collapse. The building could further collapse or start on fire. You should
    a. remove the person from danger despite other injuries and perform CPR.
    b. perform CPR in place to avoid any spinal cord injuries while restarting the heart.
    c. alternate mouth-to-mouth with CPR while stabilizing the building.
    d. wait until the victim is unconscious and then perform mouth-to-mouth in place.

47. At an archeological dig, scientists found the remains of an unknown plant no longer existing on Earth. It was discovered in the same layer as an animal whose time on Earth has already been established from previous digs and excavations.
    If this plant is found in deeper layers, it would tend to support the hypothesis that the
    a. animal also lived at the time the deeper layers existed.
    b. plant went extinct before the animal did.
    c. age of this plant can be definitively determined.
    d. age of this animal has to be determined, as it is probably older.

48. An example of sexual reproduction is
    a. budding.
    b. miotic cell division.
    c. cloning.
    d. gametes.

49. Many older trees can be completely hollow through the length of their trunk yet still be strong, healthy living trees with leaves and growth. What part of the tree makes this possible?

a. The cambium continues to grow inside the bark.

b. The shoot meristem continues to grow vertically.

c. The xylem produces new cells to increase the tree's width.

d. The phloem keeps the walls of the tree strong and supplies water.

Use the following diagram of the water cycle to answer question 50.

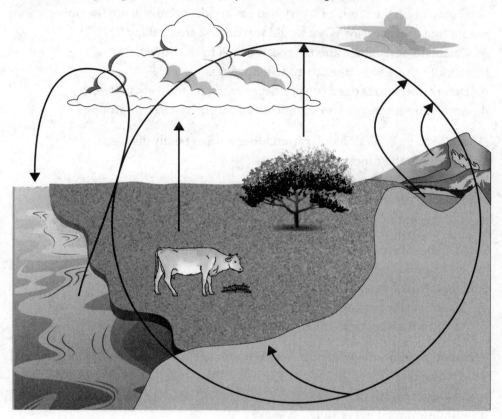

50. If the evaporation stage were not a part of the water cycle, what would happen to the cycle?

a. Water would not come up from underground as groundwater.

b. Water could not return to the atmosphere to fall again as rain or snow.

c. Rain or snow would not be able to soak into the ground.

d. Plant respiration would not occur through plant leaves.

51. A student wants to measure the amount of CO_2 she expels during both normal breathing and while she is exercising to prove that exercise increases her CO_2 output. She sets up a plastic bag to be filled with her exhalations. She then will set up a tube that will convey the contents of the exhaled air into water, bubbling up through it in a beaker. She will then measure the acidity of the water by calculating the amount of basic solution added to the water to neutralize the increased acid in the water that came from the additional CO_2 in the exhaled breath from the bag. Which step was missing from this experiment?

a. A hypothesis step where the student decides what should be measured
b. A testing step where the experiment records any changes that occur
c. A repeat step where the conditions are tested by duplicating the same results
d. A control step in which ordinary air was bubbled through water to serve as a baseline

52. You come upon the scene of a very bad car accident and you are the only person not injured in some way. What would you do first after calling 911?
a. Calculate percentage and degree of burns to the body.
b. Identify those who need to go to a hospital.
c. Determine who is dead or very near death and unlikely to live.
d. Apply direct pressure on significant bleeding that can be stopped.

53. How does drug addiction differ from other human bodily diseases?
a. It disrupts the function of an organ.
b. It can last a lifetime and kill you.
c. It can be cured without permanent effects.
d. It is preventable and is basically a brain disorder.

54. What is the difference between an amoeba and animal or plant cells?
a. An amoeba doesn't have cytoplasm.
b. An amoeba has a vacuole.
c. An amoeba is part of a multicellular organism.
d. An amoeba is a single-celled microorganism.

55. The most significant difference between animals in the phylum Chordata and other phyla is
a. bilateral symmetry.
b. a hollow dorsal nerve tube.
c. separate mouth and anus.
d. ringed specialized segments.

56. The primary function of the lymphatic system is
a. protecting the body from agents that cause disease.
b. providing for gas and heat exchange as well as sound.
c. providing for ingestion and chemical absorption.
d. transporting fluids by pumping through vessels.

57. Which fiber length reveals a skeletal type of muscle tissue?
a. 100 to 200 cm
b. 100 microns to 30 cm
c. 50 to 100 microns
d. 20 to 500 microns

58. What is one of the primary roles of mitochondria?

    a. To produce proteins
    b. To surround cytoplasm
    c. To house DNA and genes
    d. To produce ATP

59. In addition to water (H_2O), which of the following is a waste product of cellular respiration in animals?
    a. CO_2
    b. O_2
    c. O_3
    d. N_2

60. During osmosis,
    a. water molecules move through a barrier to a high concentration solution.
    b. water molecules diffuse throughout a solution to maintain stasis.
    c. a cell uses energy and physically moves a molecule through a barrier.
    d. a cell allows a release of water vapor from inside a cell into the atmosphere.

Answer Key

Practice Test 1
Verbal Ability Word Knowledge

1. **The answer is d.** The key words are *accepted* and *modes*. Only choice d describes these.

2. **The answer is c.** To emulate is to copy or imitate.

3. **The answer is a.** To deny contact is to exclude, or ostracize.

4. **The answer is a.** *Anti-* means "against," or "opposite."

5. **The answer is d.** A rendezvous is a place designated for a meeting.

6. **The answer is b.** To inhabit is to live within. A habitable home can be lived in.

7. **The answer is c.** *Fortuitous* has the same root as *fortune*.

8. **The answer is a.** *Solvent* and *dissolve* share a root.

9. **The answer is d.** *Benign* is the opposite of *malignant*.

10. **The answer is b.** Only a natural would have an affinity; an expert could learn the required skills.

11. **The answer is a.** An aimless movement would be meandering.

12. **The answer is b.** Only *brusque* suggests curt and abrupt.

13. **The answer is a.** A compact is two things coming together, as in a covenant or agreement.

14. **The answer is b.** A debacle (choice a) is a disaster, a fetish (choice c) is an obsession, and an iconoclast (choice d) describes a revolutionary or individualist.

15. **The answer is a.** The suffix *ir-* means *not,* or in this case something that cannot be revoked or that is permanent.

16. **The answer is a.** An idiom is a phrase, such as "elbow grease," that has its own special meaning.

Reading Comprehension

Passage 1

17. **The answer is b.** Choice b focuses on the disease as a whole. The varicella-zoster virus (choice a) is only the cause. The other choices just present details.

18. **The answer is c.** Fever is not mentioned among shingles symptoms.

19. **The answer is d.** Preventing the disease avoids all other treatments.

20. **The answer is a.** When someone's immune system is compromised, the virus may emerge from its dormant state.

21. **The answer is d.** The other choices are not that unusual as effects of a disease.

22. **The answer is b.** The author would advocate vaccination to avoid cost and pain.

Passage 2

23. **The answer is c.** The article is focused on cosmetics in the ancient world and their dangers to users.

24. **The answer is b.** The article states in the second paragraph that the ointment was used to clear complexions.

25. **The answer is a.** People wanted beauty first without realizing the health consequences.

26. **The answer is c.** The other results are not noted directly in the passage.

27. **The answer is d.** Blush is not specifically mentioned, although adding color to the cheeks is noted.

28. **The answer is c.** Despite this history, manufacturers want to sell their products, so the FDA must be vigilant and pull products that might be dangerous.

Passage 3

29. **The answer is d.** Only choice d expresses the larger issues the article addresses.

30. **The answer is a.** The other choices are far more active or involve force.

31. **The answer is c.** Historically, PE only was a brief exercise period. The other choices are not unique to the past.

32. **The answer is b.** Sweat is associated with hard work.

33. **The answer is c**. The definition of physical fitness has been expanded to the other choices, but not disease prevention.

34. **The answer is b**. Buschner is an expert; therefore, his opinion is highly qualified.

Passage 4

35. **The answer is d**. The article says the woolly flying squirrel hasn't been seen since 1924, not that it is extinct. If it were extinct, it would not have been found again.

36. **The answer is c**. Only this choice notes both the squirrel and its relationship to the theory.

37. **The answer is a**. The story of the woolly flying squirrel supports McKinnon's ideas about rediscovered species.

38. **The answer is c**. A stable climate means that animals need not migrate or leave. There is no support in the passage for any other answer choice.

39. **The answer is c**. The third paragraph is a narrative that tells the beginning of Zahler's story of the discovery, and it is told in a chronological sequence.

40. **The answer is d**. Choice d has nothing to do with McKinnon's regulations, so that is the correct choice.

Passage 5

41. **The answer is a**. George Thomson (choice b) was J.J. Thomson's son, and his work followed that of his father. Hertz and Lenard (choices c and d) are described as working with waves but not as particles. Of the choices, only Johnstone-Stoney is mentioned as having described the particle he called the *electron*.

42. **The answer is c**. The fact that the charge could not be removed from the rays indicated that it was a property of the particles.

43. **The answer is b**. Corpuscles are mentioned as a term of Isaac Newton's, which he used to describe particles of light long before his theories were proved. The same term was used by Thomson to describe the particles he found in cathode rays.

44. **The answer is b**. The author never goes so far as to imply that the discovery could never have been made by a single scientist (choice c), only that it was not.

45. **The answer is a**. The author calls J.J. Thomson's experiments "elegant" and credits him with determining "the existence of a subatomic particle with a negative charge."

46. **The answer is d.** A definition connecting wave-particle duality to quantum mechanics (choice d) would support the author's statement.

Word Knowledge

47. **The answer is a.** The doctor gave up on, or rejected responsibility for, her patient.

48. **The answer is d.** If public opinion is oscillating, it is shifting and changing, and polling results would then show this by fluctuating.

49. **The answer is b.** "Amor" in Latin means love, and sighing and blushing are signs of love.

50. **The answer is d.** Lassitude is extreme listlessness or weariness.

51. **The answer is c.** Something orthodox is conventional or adhering to orthodoxy, so something unorthodox is unconventional.

52. **The answer is d.** A *foster* parent, for example, raises or nurtures a child.

53. **The answer is a.** A recluse *closes* herself away from others.

54. **The answer is a.** Look for the choice that is the opposite of *innocent*.

55. **The answer is b.** Mastication is the act of chewing or grinding.

56. **The answer is b.** *Cognition* refers to knowing, and the prefix *in-* means "without." If the prince dressed incognito, he dressed so that others were without knowledge of his true identity.

57. **The answer is c.** Feelings of resentment would cause problems between employees.

58. **The answer is b.** A knoll is a small hill that something could be built "on."

59. **The answer is c.** *Placid* means calm, so placating is calming.

60. **The answer is c.** To refute is to contradict or deny, so something irrefutable is undeniable.

Mathematics

1. **The answer is d.** There are an infinite number of fractions between any two integers.

2. **The answer is d.** When an exponent is raised to an exponent, multiply them to simplify. Use the expression $4 \times 5 = 20$. Therefore, the correct answer is x^{20}.

3. **The answer is b**. First, you can convert 15:40 to a fraction and reduce it. $\frac{15}{40}$ becomes $\frac{3}{8}$, which is equal to 37.5%. This is a great one to have memorized so that you do not have to worry about the math on the actual test.

4. **The answer is d**. This problem is basic translation, but be careful with "three years younger"; it can be tricky to tell when you need to subtract.

5. **The answer is b**. To convert Fahrenheit to Celsius, subtract 32 and then multiply by $\frac{5}{9}$. $(90 - 32) \times \frac{5}{9} = 32\frac{2}{9}$, or approximately 32.

6. **The answer is a**. Because the two drawings are made from a complete deck of cards, the two events are independent of one another. We first need to determine the probability of drawing a face card of any suit from a deck of cards. Out of a total of 52 cards, there are 3 face cards of any suit and a total of 12 face cards. The probability of drawing a face card of any suit, P(A), is $\frac{12}{52}$. Because the first card is replaced before the second drawing, the probability of drawing a face card of any suit, P(B), is also $\frac{12}{52}$. Thus, the probability of drawing two face cards of the same suit is: P(A and B) = P(A) · P(b) = $\frac{12}{52} \cdot \frac{12}{52} = \frac{144}{2,704} = \frac{9}{169}$.

7. **The answer is c**. Examine the digits in the tenths place. Zero tenths is less than 2 tenths or 7 tenths, and 1.1 has a digit in the ones place, so .084 is the smallest decimal in the list.

8. **The answer is c**. $7 \times 55 = 385$, so $\frac{385}{7} = 55$.

9. **The answer is c**. Align digits by their place values and add.

10. **The answer is b**. Translate: "One dollar more than half its normal price" when the normal price is 15 translates into $\frac{1}{2} \times 15 + 1$, which is the same as choice b.

11. **The answer is d**. The mean of a data set is the sum of the values of the data set divided by the number of values or:

$$\frac{94+71+68+83+80+86+76+86+91+97+88+77+85+70+78}{15} = \frac{1,230}{15} = 82.$$

12. **The answer is b**. The median is the middle or center value of the data set when arranged in numerical order, or 83.

13. **The answer is a**. Because the integers are negative, the largest integer is –8.

14. **The answer is d**. If there are three black cars to every two white, then blacks cars represent $\frac{3}{5}$ of the cars in the parking lot. This fraction is equal to 60%, and 60% of 360 (the number of degrees in a circle) is equal to 216.

15. **The answer is d.** First, you have to determine that each child gets three cookies, because a package of six cookies is split between two children. If each child gets three cookies, that is the left side of our proportion: three cookies over one child. The right fraction is x over 12 children. Cross multiply and you get $x = 36$.

16. **The answer is a.** $5 \times 118 = 590$ and $590 + 3 = 593$, so $\frac{593}{5} = 118$ r3.

17. **The answer is c.** By multiplying the total number of contestants (250) by 0.40 you will determine that 100 runners finished the race. If 250 started it, that means 150 never finished.

18. **The answer is b.** If you are starting from about 5,000 and going to about 2,500, that is a decrease of about 2,500, which is a decrease of about $\frac{2,500}{5,000}$, or 50%.

19. **The answer is c.** The inventory of sharps increased from about 4,000 to about 5,000 during that period, so if 500 were *discarded*, a total of 1,500 must have been added to replace them and increase the inventory by 1,000.

20. **The answer is b.** Translate: $x = 2 \times 10 - 3$. Solve and you have 17.

21. **The answer is c.** You can multiply the decimal divisor by 10 to make it a whole number. You must then multiply the dividend by 10 as well to maintain the equivalence to the original problem. $\frac{3.4}{0.2} = \frac{34}{2} = 17$.

22. **The answer is b.** In order to solve the equation $10 + 5x^2 = 135$ for x, you need to isolate

$x:$ $x^2 = 135 - 10 = 125$

$x^2 = \frac{125}{2} = 25$

Taking the square root of each side of the equation yields $x = \pm 5$.

23. **The answer is b.** By multiplying 110 by 2.2, Kurt determined that he weighed 242 lbs.

24. **The answer is a.** Align digits by their place values and then subtract.

25. **The answer is c.** Multiply 782 by 1 and then by 20. Add partial products to determine that the product is 16,422.

26. **The answer is c.** This equation can be solved by simplifying each side of the equation, combining like terms, isolating x on one side of the equation, and then solving for x:

$4(2x + 20) + 3(x - 1) = 0$

$8x + 80 + 3x - 3 = 0$

$11x + 77 = 0$

$x = -\frac{77}{11} = -7$

27. **The answer is d.** Divide both sides of the inequality by 5. $\frac{5y}{5} > \frac{6}{5}$, so $y > \frac{6}{5}$, which is equivalent to $1\frac{1}{5}$.

28. **The answer is b.** Choices b and d are the only answers that are negative, so you can eliminate choices a and c. Because 1 is a fraction between 0 and −1, 3 is not as far to the left as −3, and therefore not as small.

29. **The answer is b.** 3,498 divided by 26 gives 134.54. Disregarding the remainder, the correct choice is b.

30. **The answer is a.** You can multiply the numerator and denominator of $\frac{7}{9}$ by 4 to see that it is equivalent to $\frac{28}{36}$. You can multiply the numerator and denominator of $\frac{1}{4}$ by 9 to see that it is equivalent to $\frac{9}{36}$. Then subtract. $\frac{28}{36} - \frac{9}{36} = \frac{19}{36}$.

31. **The answer is a.** This problem can be done by comparing individual fractions, but it is probably more time consuming than the alternate, which is converting the fractions into decimals so that they are easier to order: $\frac{1}{8} = 0.125$, $\frac{2}{5} = 0.4$, $\frac{1}{2} = 0.5$ and $\frac{3}{4} = 0.75$, so that is the order they should be in from left to right.

32. **The answer is c.** The mixed number $4\frac{5}{7}$ can be converted into a fraction as follows:
$$4\frac{5}{7} = \frac{4 \cdot 7 + 5}{7} = \frac{28 + 5}{7} = \frac{33}{7}.$$

33. **The answer is d.** In total, 60 days of 200 mg per day would be 12,000 mg. Dividing this by 1,000 means 12 grams would be needed.

34. **The answer is a.** There were three days with no rainfall, whereas no other amount occurred that many days, so 0 is the mode.

35. **The answer is b.** The prime factors of 28 are 2, 2, and 7, so their sum is 11.

36. **The answer is b.** To perform the subtraction $4\frac{5}{6} - 2\frac{3}{4}$, you should first convert each of the fractions from a mixed number to its standard form and then find a common denominator to complete the subtraction process:
$$4\frac{5}{6} = \frac{4 \cdot 6 + 5}{6} = \frac{24 + 5}{6} = \frac{29}{6} \quad 2\frac{3}{4} = \frac{2 \cdot 4 + 3}{4} = \frac{8 + 3}{4} = \frac{11}{4}$$
$$4\frac{5}{6} - 2\frac{3}{4} = \frac{29}{6} - \frac{11}{4} = \frac{58 - 33}{12} = \frac{25}{12}.$$

37. **The answer is d.** As a fraction, 80% is $\frac{80}{100}$, but in its simplest form both numerator and denominator would be divided by 10 or $\frac{8}{10}$.

38. **The answer is c.** The radius of the circle is 4 in. When you plug that into the formula for circumference, you get $C = 2\pi r C = 2(4)\pi = 8\pi$.

39. **The answer is b.** The median of the ordered list -8, -1, 3, 4, and 12 is 3.

40. **The answer is b.** Ignoring the decimals, 38×235 is 8,930, and there are four digits behind the decimal in 0.38 and 2.35, so you move the decimal four places to the left to get 0.8930 or just 0.893.

Science

1. **The answer is c.** By comparing the cell type of any living thing to another, the most basic comparison is whether or not a cell has a nucleus with DNA bound in a membrane (eukaryotes) or if it lacks a cell nucleus with membrane-bound organelles (prokaryotes). The other groups shown are more distinct classifications and would not contain all living things.

2. **The answer is c.** One mole of a substance weighs its gram formula mass. Because there are two oxygen atoms (16 grams each) present, the weight is 32.0 grams per mole.

3. **The answer is a.** The three types of muscles are smooth, skeletal, and cardiac. The nerves do not need muscles to function.

4. **The answer is a.** The septum (1) is the part of the heart that separates the left and right sides. The (2) right atrium receives blood from the body, the (3) aorta delivers blood to the body, and the (4) left ventricle pumps blood to the aorta and the lungs.

5. **The answer is a.** The phylum Mollusca contains octopi and squid, which do not have shells like other members of the phylum. All members, however, have a soft body without any bones, but they do have nerves, and most have a foot or tentacles.

6. **The answer is b.** Vector quantities have both a magnitude and direction. Scalar quantities have only a magnitude.

7. **The answer is c.** This arrow shows the distance from the normal of the wave to the maximum height above the normal. This represents the amplitude of the wave.

8. **The answer is d.** Because 2 moles weigh 8.0 grams, 1 mole of the substance will weigh 4.0 grams. The weight of one mole of a substance is its gram atomic mass. This corresponds to helium, He.

9. **The answer is a.** The heart is made of muscle. This type of muscle is called cardiac muscle.

10. **The answer is c.** Tears, urine, and mucus are all primary lines of defense, because they work to prevent infection. Inflammation is an example of a second line of defense, because it works once the body has been infected.

11. **The answer is b.** The top or meniscus of the mercury column is between 100° and 101° and is very close to 101.5°.

12. **The answer is a.** This circuit is a series circuit because there is only one pathway that the current can take.

13. **The answer is d.** The volume of 1 mole of a gas at STP is 22.4 liters, and 3 moles of the gas is three times the molar volume, or 67.2 liters.

14. **The answer is c.** Vitamin D helps with the absorption of calcium so that teeth and bones can grow and develop properly.

15. **The answer is d.** The epiglottis covers the larynx so that food does not enter; this ensures that the food goes down the esophagus.

16. **The answer is a.** The diaphragm is a sheet of muscle that contracts and expands the chest cavity and assists the mechanics of breathing.

17. **The answer is c.** According to the equation $v = f\lambda$, for velocity to remain constant, if the frequency increases, then the wavelength must decrease. If the frequency decreases, then the wavelength must increase. This is an inverse relationship.

18. **The answer is c.** The gram formula mass of water is 18 grams per mole. The weight of the oxygen present makes up 16 of 18 grams per mole. Dividing 16 by 18 gives 0.888 or 88.9%.

19. **The answer is b.** Synapses are the spaces between neurons. This space allows neurotransmitters to move between the neurons.

20. **The answer is b.** The liver works to clean and detoxify the blood. The liver also produces bile, which is stored in the gallbladder.

21. **The answer is d.** Although we see water in a wave entering the pipe, the water would not turn the blade because contact with seawater would soon corrode metal parts. Instead, the moving water also forces air into the tube and pushes it up an air-venting pipe. The rush of air creates the pressure to spin a turbine both coming in and being drawn back out as the wave recedes in the tube.

22. **The answer is b.** Work is equal to force times distance, $W = Fd$.

23. **The answer is d.** The glucose is the solute and water is the solvent because the glucose changes its phase and the water does not.

24. **The answer is b.** The villi (microvilli) in the small intestine act the same way roots do, to increase the surface area so that more substances can be absorbed into the body.

25. **The answer is b.** Estrogen is a hormone produced by females. It is produced in the ovaries and not in the adrenal medulla.

26. **The answer is c.** A change in the food chain would occur first but wouldn't necessarily cause a die-off of healthy fish without an increased blood of algae, which would cause oxygen despletion in the water.

27. **The answer is a.** If an object has a constant speed, it is not accelerating. Therefore, the acceleration is zero.

28. **The answer is a.** There are 58.5 grams of NaCl in 1 mole of NaCl. Setting up to calculate the molarity of the solution, you divide 1.0 mole by 0.500 liters:

$$\frac{1.0 \text{ mole}}{0.500 \text{ liter}} = 2.0 \text{ M.}$$

29. **The answer is c.** Gases diffuse through membranes and into the blood. This happens at the capillaries located at the alveoli.

30. **The answer is d.** The central nervous system is composed of the brain and spinal cord. This is easy to remember because they lie down the center of the body.

31. **The answer is b.** Thermal energy comes from particle movement and heat. Kinetic energy describes motion and inertia. Nuclear energy comes from subatomic particles. Only potential energy describes the energy an object possesses without movement.

32. **The answer is a.** Because the cell is in a solution where the concentration of solutes is higher inside the cell than outside the cell, water is expected to flow into the cell to dilute the concentration of solutes inside the cell. This causes the cells to swell up and possibly burst.

33. **The answer is c.** Using the equation for molarity, the number of moles divided by 2.0 liters equals 1.5. If 3.0 moles are dissolved in the 2.0 liters of solution, the concentration is 1.5 M.

34. **The answer is a.** The average person in good health has a pulse of about 72 beats per minute and a blood pressure of 120 over 80 mm Hg.

35. **The answer is a.** Ligaments hold bone to bone. Tendons hold muscle to bone.

36. **The answer is a.** Avogadro's number is used to determine the number of moles there are of a substance.

37. **The answer is c.** Timbre distinguishes musical sounds with identical pitch and loudness. Tone quality characterizes the same note played by different instruments with the same loudness. Dark, warm, or harsh are other types of timbre.

38. **The answer is c.** The products of fermentation are ethanol and carbon dioxide. It is the carbon dioxide that causes the dough to rise.

39. **The answer is d.** "DNA cannot be altered" is a false statement because DNA can be mutated and changed. The other answer choices are true statements.

40. **The answer is a.** As water is evaporated from a solution, the concentration of the solute in the solution increases because there is less water present.

41. **The answer is d.** The formation of an ion depends on the loss or gain of electrons. If the ion is negative, then the ion must have gained a negatively charged electron.

42. **The answer is b.** Gases show a decrease in solubility in water with an increase in temperature. The other three choices are salts, and they show an increase in solubility as temperature increases.

43. **The answer is a.** Optic refers to the eye, where the retina is located. Olfactory refers to the nose, and auditory refers to the ear.

44. **The answer is b.** Smooth muscle is the type of muscle found in the digestive system.

45. **The answer is d.** A patient suffering from respiratory acidosis needs to increase the pH of the blood. CO_2 levels need to be lowered through ventilation.

46. **The answer is a.** In choice b, the diastolic pressure is too low relative to the systolic. In choice c, the overall pressure is too low. In choice d, the diastolic pressure is too high relative to the systolic.

47. **The answer is b.** Mitosis creates cells that are exact copies of each other, including the number of chromosomes in the cell. Meiosis, which creates sex cells, forms cells with half the number of chromosomes in the original cell.

48. **The answer is c.** The ribs are in front of the lungs in the human body, making them closer to the front of the body. This is best described as being anterior.

49. **The answer is a.** As a solute is added to a solvent, the solvent undergoes a freezing point depression and a boiling point elevation.

50. **The answer is d.** The ability of carbon to form strong bonds and long chains and to have various functional groups allows for millions of organic compounds that are essential to life.

51. **The answer is a.** The mandible is the jaw bone. The ribs are located in the chest, whereas the radius and femur are located in the arm and leg, respectively.

52. **The answer is c.** The term *renal* refers to the kidney. The term *pulmonary* refers to the lungs.

53. **The answer is d.** Choices a, b, and c are parts of the female reproductive system. The epididymis is part of the male reproductive system and lies on the testicles.

54. **The answer is a.** The iris and retina are just a few of the many parts of the eye.

55. **The answer is a.** Melting is the phase transition from solid to liquid. The phase diagram with the regions labeled is shown below. Only the transitions from A to B would include melting when the substance crosses the solid-liquid line.

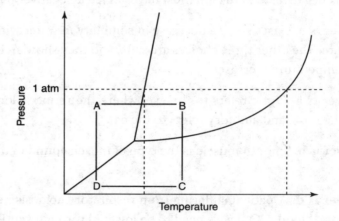

56. **The answer is b.** The raising and lowering of the diaphragm causes the inside of the chest cavity to expand, and with a larger space in the lungs, outside air pressure flows in to achieve equilibrium. If the larynx is constricted, air could not flow. The ribs extend, the muscles of the rib cage expand and contract, while the capacity of the lungs actually increases during respiration.

57. **The answer is b.** Sphincters help keep food in the stomach while it is being digested, and the anus is a sphincter that prevents fecal matter from being eliminated until the organism is ready to do so.

58. **The answer is a.** The heart and veins have valves to ensure that the blood flows in only one direction.

59. **The answer is b.** The molecule has four carbon atoms in a straight chain that are joined by single bonds. This is called butane.

60. **The answer is c.** This is a five carbon, straight chain, which contains a double bond. The double bond makes it classified as an alkene.

Practice Test 2

Verbal Ability Word Knowledge

1. **The answer is a.** Someone who is altruistic is generous.

2. **The answer is b.** Compensation is recompense for the work the explorers did.

3. **The answer is c.** Something that is fraudulent and doubtable is bogus.

4. **The answer is d.** In Greek, *homo* means "one," or in this case, the same, or uniform.

5. **The answer is b.** Someone who makes you double-check is careful.

6. **The answer is c.** Think of vessels in the circulatory system.

7. **The answer is b.** Coming and going is off-and-on, or sporadic, not chronic (choice c) or consistent (choice d).

8. **The answer is a.** Someone who is new would be nervy or audacious to speak with temerity.

9. **The answer is a.** If they are not loyal, they are disloyal, or perfidious.

10. **The answer is c.** The prefix *ex-* means "out" or "to get out."

11. **The answer is b.** Read between the lines to understand that using candor is speaking your mind.

12. **The answer is a.** To alleviate pressure is to ease or lessen it.

13. **The answer is d.** Look to *unstable* and *precipice*, and you can see that the situation is dangerous or precarious.

14. **The answer is c.** A salute is an act of greeting or acknowledgment, as is a salutation in a letter.

15. **The answer is c.** A pariah is an exile or outsider, especially one who is shunned by insiders.

16. **The answer is d.** To dispute is to debate or quarrel with—to contradict.

Reading Comprehension

Passage 1

17. **The answer is d.** The focus of the entire article is the need for sleep for children.

18. **The answer is a.** This is a detail noted in the article. Choices b and c are mentioned as times when children actually sleep less.

19. **The answer is b.** Questionnaires are mentioned in paragraph 3.

20. **The answer is d.** The article notes all the other details but not anorexia.

21. **The answer is b.** This conclusion is the only one that is neither countered by the text nor stretched beyond the limits of the text.

22. **The answer is c.** The author states that this information "is still not clear" and "needs to be explored."

Passage 2

23. **The answer is c.** Ether's run is described as "brief but important," implying that despite its short reign as the anesthetic of choice, it was an effective choice.

24. **The answer is b.** The passage really focuses on a single anesthetic, not a variety of them as choices a or c would indicate.

25. **The answer is d.** Only choice d does not fit; it states only that the usefulness of ether had not been discovered for many years.

26. **The answer is a.** "Supposed to have discovered" means that Lullus is "said to have discovered." It implies that there is not a lot of corroborating evidence; if there were, the author would have simply said "discovered."

27. **The answer is c.** The fourth paragraph is a narrative that tells about Morton's demonstration, followed by his attempts to win a patent. It is told in story form, in the order in which events occurred.

28. **The answer is a.** Long performed an operation using ether before Morton did.

Passage 3

29. **The answer is c.** Refining is one of the three steps in the creation of aluminum.

30. **The answer is c.** According to the third paragraph, "Bulldozers remove the topsoil, and excavators or other types of power machinery are used to remove the underlying layer of bauxite."

31. **The answer is c.** The fourth paragraph describes the process of refinement and its by-products. Those that are mentioned in the paragraph include choices a, b, and d. There is no mention of choice c, which is an alloy of aluminum and an element not involved in this refining process.

32. **The answer is a.** A quick scan of the third, fourth, and fifth paragraphs indicates that all three are steps in the process of making aluminum.

33. **The answer is b.** The mention of protests indicates that working people are beginning to question the dangers of mining.

34. **The answer is a.** In the final paragraph, the author states, "As with all mining of metals, bauxite mining presents certain hazards."

Passage 4

35. **The answer is c.** The passage focuses on the promise of acupuncture alone.

36. **The answer is a.** Side effects mean there is no entirely safe treatment for menstrual cramps.

37. **The answer is b.** Pain is pain, and what worked with one pain could work with another type.

38. **The answer is c.** Less risk is always a main advantage.

39. **The answer is d.** The passage concludes that acupuncture is useful for this condition.

40. **The answer is b.** The widespread use of acupuncture suggests it would have a variety of practical uses beyond those for whom it is now accepted practice.

Passage 5

41. **The answer is b.** The article focuses on cosmetic procedures, not on the lesser issues stated.

42. **The answer is b.** Cosmetic surgery is intended to make someone more attractive.

43. **The answer is d.** Liposuction is the most popular, but of the procedures on this list, breast augmentation is the most popular.

44. **The answer is c.** Men want to stop the aging process and defeat wrinkles.

45. **The answer is c.** Men are not so different when it comes to making themselves more attractive.

46. **The answer is d.** The other choices do not derive logically from the passage.

Word Knowledge

47. **The answer is b.** Lacking training, she would need to be intuitive.

48. **The answer is a.** Choosing not to perform an operation would draw attention, or examination.

49. **The answer is d.** People tried but failed, making the result something that could not be prevented.

50. **The answer is c.** To placate someone is to calm them down.

51. **The answer is b.** To engender a feeling of discontent is to cause or generate that feeling.

52. **The answer is c.** When wind, rain, and abrasion cause erosion, they break down rock. When a relationship erodes, it breaks down.

53. **The answer is b.** They were admired because they performed under difficult conditions. The key word *despite* indicates that they performed well in the face of something that might ordinarily cause them to perform badly.

54. **The answer is d.** *Port* in Latin indicates something carried, as in *report* or *transport*. A rumor may be carried in this way.

55. **The answer is a.** When something bears fruit, it is successfully completed.

56. **The answer is b.** Someone sagacious is very wise, and someone imprudent is rash and unwise.

57. **The answer is a.** Consider how the word is commonly used: "Ted had an affinity for music." He was attracted to it, or felt a kinship with it.

58. **The answer is c.** Try the other words in the sentence, and none fits with the idea of cutting costs.

59. **The answer is c.** Harry did not like the macabre, or gruesome, nature of haunted houses.

60. **The answer is d.** The opposite of *opulent*, or *lavish*, is *simple*.

Mathematics

1. **The answer is a.** To divide 2.4×10^6 by -1.2×10^3, first arrange in the proper form of division and then separately divide the coefficients and the exponents:

$$\frac{2.4}{-1.2} \times \frac{10^6}{10^3} = -2 \times 10^3$$

2. **The answer is b.** To determine the product of 3.2 and 4.16, the numbers should be arranged as:

$$
\begin{array}{r}
4.16 \\
\times\ 3.2 \\
\hline
832 \\
1{,}248 \\
\hline
13.312
\end{array}
$$

3. **The answer is b.** In scientific notation, the number 13.9 is 1.39×10^1.

4. **The answer is c.** To find the total number of girls in the science class, we must first find the fraction of students in the class who are girls. For every set of 5 students, 2 students are girls, yielding a fraction of $\frac{2}{5}$. Thus, the total number of girls in the class is $\frac{2}{5} \times 430 = 172$.

5. **The answer is c.** The quotient of $(6x^2y^5z^3)$ divided by $3x^2y^3z^6$ or $\frac{6x^2y^5z^3}{3x^2y^3z^6}$ can be found by:

$$\frac{6x^2y^5z^3}{3x^2y^3z^6} = \frac{6}{3} \times \frac{x^2}{x^2} \times \frac{y^5}{y^3} \times \frac{z^3}{z^6} = 2 \times 1 \times y^2 \times \frac{1}{z^3} = \frac{2y^3}{z^3}.$$

6. **The answer is d.** Simplifying the expression in terms of its factors,

$$\frac{x^2 + x - 42}{x + 7} = \frac{(x+7)(x-6)}{x+7} = x - 6 = 1. \text{ Solving for } x \text{ yields } 6 + 1 = 7.$$

7. **The answer is c.** By converting $\frac{2}{3}$ to a decimal, or 0.67, and multiplying 7.67 by 0.13, the cost would be $0.997, or $1.00.

8. **The answer is c.** Set up a proportion of the unknown percentage over 100 with the known percentage of $\frac{1,140}{920}$. Divide the denominator by the numerator.

9. **The answer is b.** Ten decimeters multiplied by 10 centimeters is 100 centimeters in a meter, so by dividing 435 by 100, there are 4.35 meters in 435 centimeters.

10. **The answer is b.** Create top-heavy fractions with the same denominators to allow simple subtraction of $\frac{21}{3} = \frac{11}{3} = \frac{10}{3}$ or $3\frac{1}{3}$.

11. **The answer is c.** Multiply $\frac{38}{1} \times \frac{7}{16}$, then simplify by dividing the numerator and denominator by 2 to get $\frac{133}{8}$.

12. **The answer is d.** Set up a proportion:

$$\frac{1}{4} = \frac{x}{1,890,000}$$

$4x = 1,890,000$

$x = 472,500$

13. **The answer is a.** Both the spinning and yoga classes have seen participation go up over both years.

14. **The answer is a.** Spinning saw an increase of 5 from 2006 to 2007.

15. **The answer is c.** $(12 + 5 + 1 + 0 + 7) \div 5 = 5$.

16. **The answer is d.** $769 + 351 = 1,120$.

17. **The answer is b.** This is a proportion problem, so you can set up two equal fractions: 75 cents and 1 shirt on the left, and 1,500 cents and x on the right. Cross-multiply and you get $75x = 1,500$. Divide each side by 75 and you $x = 20$.

18. **The answer is d.** To convert Celsius to Fahrenheit, multiply by $\frac{9}{5}$ and then add 32. $60 \times \frac{9}{5} + 32 = 108 + 32$, so the answer is 140°F.

19. **The answer is c.** The prime factors of 75 are 3, 5, and 5, giving you a sum of 13.

20. **The answer is b.** Be careful to subtract not add.

21. **The answer is a.** Dividing means subtracting exponents, so $\frac{y^7}{y^4}$ is the same as y^{7-4}, or y^3.

22. **The answer is a.** You may have noticed that since 27 can only go into 78 twice, the answer must be 29.

23. **The answer is c.** Translate: $x = 0.6 \times 60$. Multiplying it out gives you $x = 36$, or choice c.

24. **The answer is c.** Set up a basic proportion with 45 (cents) over 2 (holes) on the left and x over 10 (holes) on the right. Then you can cross-multiply to get $45 \times 10 = 2x$ and solve to get $225 = x$. Of course, you then need to express that in dollars to fit the answer choices, and 225 cents = $2.25.

25. **The answer is c.** The problem asks for the area of a triangle, so you need to plug the numbers you are given into the formula for the area of a triangle, $A = \frac{1}{2bh}$, giving you $A = \frac{1}{2} \times 10 \times 9$, which solves to $A = 45$ in².

26. **The answer is b.** The formula for area of a circle is $A = \pi r^2$, so plugging the radius 4 into the formula gives $A = \pi 4^2$ or $A = 16\pi$.

27. **The answer is b.** $\frac{7}{8}$ divides out as 0.875, so choice b is the correct answer.

28. **The answer is a.** This equation $x^2 - 7x - 18 = 0$ can be solved using the quadratic formula; however, it can also be factored: $(x - 9)(x + 2) = x^2 - 7x - 18$, so $x = 9$ and $x = -2$.

$x = \dfrac{-b \pm \sqrt{b^2 - 4ac}}{2a}$, where $a = 1$, $b = -7$, and $c = -18$. Substituting into the formula yields:

$x = \dfrac{-(-7) \pm \sqrt{(-7^2) - 4(1)(-18)}}{2(1)} = \dfrac{7 \pm \sqrt{49 + 72}}{2} = \dfrac{7 \pm \sqrt{121}}{2} = \dfrac{7 \pm 11}{2}$.

The roots of the quadratic equation are: $x = \dfrac{7 + 11}{2} = \dfrac{18}{2} = 9$ and $x = \dfrac{7 - 11}{2} = \dfrac{-4}{2} = -2$.

29. **The answer is b.** The product of $(4a^2b^4c)$ and $(-7a^5b^3)$ can be found by:

$$(4a^2b^4c) \times (x - 7a^5b^3) = (4x - 7) \times (a^2 \times a^5) \times (b^4 \times b^3) \times (c \times 1) = -28 \times a^7 \times b^7 \times c = -28a^7b^7c.$$

30. **The answer is c.** The sum of the polynomials, $5x + 3xy - 6y^2$, $9xy + 7y^2 - 4x$, and $-8y^2 + 7x + 12xy$ can be found by combining like terms. Simplifying the expression yields:

$$5x - 4x + 7x + 3xy + 9xy + 12xy - 6y^2 + 7y^2 - 8y^2 = 8x + 24xy - 7y^2.$$

31. **The answer is c.** Because the base is common, the product is obtained by simply adding the exponents and calculating the result or $3^3 \cdot 3^2 \cdot 3^1 = 3^{3+2+1} = 3^6 = 729$.

32. **The answer is d.** The roots of a quadratic equation $3x^2 - x - 10 = 0$ can be found by factoring—$3x^2 - x - 10 = (3x + 5)(x - 2)$ so the roots are $x = -5/3$ and $x = 2$—or by using the quadratic formula: $\dfrac{-b \pm \sqrt{b^2 - 4ac}}{2a}$, where $a = 3$, $b = -1$, and $c = -10$. Substituting into the formula yields: $x = \dfrac{-(-1) \pm \sqrt{(-1)^2 - 4(3)(-10)}}{2(3)} =$

$\dfrac{1 \pm \sqrt{1 + 120}}{6} = \dfrac{1 \pm \sqrt{121}}{6} = \dfrac{1 \pm 11}{6}$, yielding the roots $x = \dfrac{1+11}{6} = \dfrac{12}{6} = 2$ and $x = \dfrac{1-11}{6} = \dfrac{-10}{6} = \dfrac{5}{3}$.

33. **The answer is c.** There are three feet to a yard, so to convert a meter to feet, multiply 1.094 by 3, which equals 3.282 feet.

34. **The answer is d.** Multiply $4x$ by $2x$ first for $8x^2$. Then multiply $4x$ by 4 for $16x$ and -2 by $2x$ to get $-4x$. Add these together for $12x$. Complete with $-2 \times 4 = -8$.

35. **The answer is d.** In each restatement of the problem, each equation maintained equality on both sides of the equal sign.

36. **The answer is a.** Create an equation that restates the conditions. The first number would be $1x$. Added to the second number it would be $1x + \dfrac{3}{5x}$ and their total would be divided by 2 to make

$$20: \dfrac{1x + \dfrac{3}{5}x}{2} = 20$$

Multiply both sides by 2: $1x + \dfrac{3}{5}x = 40$

Convert $1x$ to like form: $\dfrac{5}{5x} + \dfrac{3}{5}x = 40$

Add the fractions: $\dfrac{8}{5x} = 40$

Multiply both sides by $5x$.

$8 = 200x$

$x = 25$

37. **The answer is d**. The fraction $\frac{60}{12}$ divides out to 5, which is the same as 500%.

38. **The answer is c**. There are 100 centimeters in a meter, so there are 56×100, or 5,600 centimeters in 56 meters.

39. **The answer is b**. If Jane has collected 132 stamps over 12 months, she has collected an average of 132 stamps over 12 months, she has collected an average of $132 \div 12 = 11$ stamps per month.

40. **The answer is a**. When you convert $2\frac{66}{84}$ into an improper fraction, you get $\frac{234}{84}$. Divide both numerator and denominator by 6 to get $\frac{39}{14}$.

Science

1. **The answer is c**. The Latin prefix *photo-* means "light." Plants will adjust their stem to position themselves to receive as much sunlight as possible.

2. **The answer is d**. Algae produces large amounts of food for herbivores to eat. In doing so, it supports a wide variety of consumers, many of whom are preyed upon by carnivores.

3. **The answer is a**. Using dyes and a fluoroscope, an angiogram creates of portrait of blood flow. An electroencephalogram measures electrical activity in the brain, while an echogram uses sound to detect abnormalities. Amniocentesis is a test of the health of a fetus during pregnancy.

4. **The answer is c**. An ecosystem describes a relationship with living things and their environment. Depending on the scope being considered, an ecosystem could be as broad as a biome or as limited as a pond site, and often more than one ecosystem overlaps another.

5. **The answer is b**. An ionic bond involves a change in charge because one element gives up one or more electrons and other takes them. Covalent bonds share electrons in various ways.

6. **The answer is c**. A low pH in the stomach, cilia present in the trachea, and mucus present in the nasal cavity are primary defenses. Cells within the body recognizing a pathogen are a third line of defense.

7. **The answer is a**. The movement of air through the respiratory system depends on the movements of the diaphragm. It is the movement of this muscle that creates a void space, allowing air to rush in.

8. **The answer is a**. Sperm are produced in the testes, stored in the epididymis, and then travel through the vas deferens and urethra.

9. **The answer is d.** Cartilage is a soft type of bone that lacks rigidity. This is why you are able to bend your ears.

10. **The answer is a.** The autonomic nervous system guides the actions of organs and involuntary muscles. However, because involuntary muscles are involved, you cannot control those actions.

11. **The answer is d.** The ureter, although part of the excretory system, is not part of the kidney.

12. **The answer is a.** An amino acid has an amine and a carboxylic acid group present. These are represented by $R-NH_2$ and $R-COOH$.

13. **The answer is a.** Organic chemistry is the study of carbon.

14. **The answer is c.** Blue litmus paper turns red when the pH of a solution is acidic. The number 6 corresponds to this type of pH.

15. **The answer is d.** A salt and H_2 gas form when an acid reacts with an active metal.

16. **The answer is d.** $HC_2H_3O_2$ is acetic acid, the major ingredient in vinegar. It is an acid and tastes sour, the way citric acid can make lemons taste sour.

17. **The answer is c.** The reactions are labeled as shown below:

    $$^{232}_{90}\text{Th} \rightarrow {}^{228}_{88}\text{Ra} + {}^{4}_{2}\text{He} \qquad\qquad \text{Nuclear decay}$$

    $$\text{NaCl} + H_2O \rightarrow \text{HCl} + \text{NaOH} \qquad \text{Hydrolysis (opposite of neutralization)}$$

    $$2\text{HNO}_3 + \text{Mg(OH)}_2 \rightarrow 2H_2O + \text{Mg(NO}_3)_2 \quad \text{Neutralization}$$

    $$\text{CH}_4 + 2\text{O}_2 \rightarrow \text{CO}_2 + 2H_2O \qquad\qquad \text{Combustion}$$

18. **The answer is a.** Although many anatomical structures contain valves, the bicuspid valve is located in the human heart.

19. **The answer is d.** Accessory organs aid other organs. In this case, the liver, pancreas, and gallbladder all aid the organs of the digestive system by secreting digestive juices into the digestive tract. The stomach is part of the digestive tract and does not fall under the category of accessory organ.

20. **The answer is c.** Bile is produced in the liver and is stored in the gallbladder. The function of bile is to emulsify fats, allowing them to be easily absorbed and digested by the small intestine.

21. **The answer is a.** When a solute is added to a solvent, the boiling point increases and the freezing point decreases.

22. **The answer is b**. The equation $P = IV$, power equals current times voltage, is the equation to use. Dividing the power by voltage gives $I = \dfrac{P}{V}$, and $\dfrac{60\,\text{watts}}{110\,\text{volts}}$ is 0.55 amperes.

23. **The answer is a**. Posterior refers to being behind. The kidneys are behind the small intestine.

24. **The answer is b**. Enzymes can be identified by the ending *-ase*. Proteases are enzymes that digest proteins.

25. **The answer is c**. Antibodies, killer T cells, and phagocytes all work to destroy foreign invaders in human bodies. Viruses are an example of these invaders.

26. **The answer is d**. The diaphragm is the muscle that moves to create a void in the chest. This allows air to rush through the respiratory system and fill the void created.

27. **The answer is d**. White blood cells are produced in the bone marrow and not by the skin.

28. **The answer is a**. Although all four choices are associated with the nerve cell, the synapse is not an actual part of the nerve cell. Instead, the synapse is a gap between nerve cells in which neurotransmitters move from one nerve cell to another.

29. **The answer is d**. Metals can be reshaped without losing their properties because their electron clusters can form and reform in a variety of ways without losing their structure. Ionic crystalline structures would break.

30. **The answer is c**. A pH reading of 2 would have a hydrogen ion concentration of 1×10^{-2} M and be considered acidic.

31. **The answer is d**. Refraction is the bending of light that takes place as light travels from one medium into another. It occurs because of the change in speed of the light.

32. **The answer is d**. The far more numerous rods define general shades of light and function best in low-light conditions but leave colors and bright-light conditions to the far fewer cones.

33. **The answer is d**. Kinetic energy comes from movement, so reducing the volume or temperature of a gas will change the movement of its molecules. Collisions between molecules, elastic collisions, however, result in no energy gain or loss.

34. **The answer is b**. The fallopian tubes conduct eggs to the uterus for fertilization through the vagina.

35. **The answer is c**. The purpose of the endocrine systems is to release hormones (chemical signals) into the body to regulate the body's functions.

36.   **The answer is c.** Plant cells are different from animal cells because plant cells have cell walls and contain chloroplasts to carry out photosynthesis.

37.   **The answer is b.** The roots of a plant are not responsible for carrying out photosynthesis. This is the job of the chloroplasts.

38.   **The answer is c.** Red and blue light are best absorbed by chlorophyll. This corresponds to wavelengths of 660 nm and 430 nm, respectively.

39.   **The answer is a.** The stamen is considered to be a male part of the plant reproductive system, whereas the pistil, stigma, and style (and ovary) are considered to be female parts of the plant reproductive system.

40.   **The answer is b.** A pH of 3 is one thousands times as strong as a pH of 6 because the pH scale works on powers of 10. Three pH units means a difference of 10^3 or 1,000 times.

41.   **The answer is c.** A basic solution has fewer hydronium ions and more hydroxide ions.

42.   **The answer is c.** Because the powdered magnesium has a greater surface area, it reacts faster than one solid strip of magnesium.

43.   **The answer is a.** Because water can dilute a solution, adding water lowers the concentration of the substances. This would cause the reactants to react slowly. Instead, it would have been better to mix the reactants directly.

44.   **The answer is a.** Transverse waves do not have areas of compression and expansion as they move perpendicular to the direction of the wave.

45.   **The answer is b.** According to the equation, $v = f\lambda$, the frequency is equal to the velocity of the wave divided by the wavelength. Dividing 20 m/s by 4 m gives 5 s^{-1}.

46.   **The answer is c.** Because of its smooth surface, the angle of incidence is expected to be equal to the angle of reflection.

47.   **The answer is c.** Dispersion is the breaking up of white light into the colors of the rainbow.

48.   **The answer is c.** The other name for the digestive system is the alimentary canal. One mnemonic device to remember is that the word *aliment* is French for *food*.

49.   **The answer is c.** A vector quantity has both a magnitude and a direction. A scalar quantity has only a magnitude.

50.   **The answer is a.** Only choice a has both a direction and magnitude, making it a vector.

51.   **The answer is d.** The velocity is the change in distance over time. This object went 100 m in 10 s, making the velocity 10 m/s.

52. **The answer is a**. Velocity = distance/time. Rearranging the equation, distance is equal to time multiplied by velocity. This gives: (15 m/s)(5 s) = 75 m.

53. **The answer is b**. An object that has a constant velocity does not experience any acceleration because there is no change in the velocity, a component needed to calculate acceleration.

54. **The answer is b**. The rounded atomic mass of carbon is 12; therefore, it would make up 27% or $\frac{12}{44} \times 100\%$ of the total formula mass.

55. **The answer is b**. Energy in the form of sugar is carried in specialized tissue from the leaves. Water is brought from the roots in other tissue called xylem. Oxygen is released through the leaves in cellular respiration.

56. **The answer is c**. As photosynthesis occurs, the amount of oxygen produced in the test tube will increase, affecting the volume in the test tube. The other factors are controls.

57. **The answer is d**. Number 4, the mitochondria, are the organelles responsible for energy production in the cell. The nucleolus (1) makes ribosomal ribonucleic acid (rRNA) needed to produce ribosomes. The Golgi apparatus (2) modifies and repackages proteins and lipids and sends them throughout the cell. The cell membrane (3) is a selectively permeable barrier between the cell and its external environment.

58. **The answer is d**. The optic nerve emerges from the back of the eye, opposite the opening to the light.

59. **The answer is b**. The cornea covers the opening into the eye and protects it, but it does not have any blood vessels so it can remain crystal clear and emit light only.

60. **The answer is c**. The dedicated purpose of a red blood cell is to carry oxygen so its total volume is nearly all hemoglobin and enzymes. Leukocytes are white blood cells.

Practice Test 3
Verbal Ability Word Knowledge

1. **The answer is b**. His milieu is his typical cultural and social setting.

2. **The answer is d**. In Greek, *neo-* means "new," and a novice is one who is just beginning.

3. **The answer is b**. To take umbrage is to take offense.

4. **The answer is c.** *Vociferous* comes from the same root as *vocal*; the lawyer, unlike her client, was loud, or strident.

5. **The answer is c.** To *forbode* is to indicate beforehand, especially to indicate something bad.

6. **The answer is d.** To incise something (choice a) is to cut it cleanly; a laceration is a jagged cut.

7. **The answer is b.** A blight is something that ruins or destroys.

8. **The answer is b.** She would not want to ignore (choice a) or facilitate (choice c) such a problem, she would want to curtail, or reduce, it.

9. **The answer is a.** High costs can prohibit spending—they are prohibitive.

10. **The answer is a.** To do something surreptitiously is to do it in a secretive way.

11. **The answer is b.** Not cashing in something for money indicates gross indifference.

12. **The answer is a.** A secret has to be kept private and not shared in a showy manner. Someone who is discreet is restrained and cautious about sharing.

13. **The answer is c.** Sedition is subversive, rebellious behavior.

14. **The answer is b.** "Some" radiation indicates that it wasn't a huge amount.

15. **The answer is d.** To be in flux is to be fluctuating, or flowing back and forth.

16. **The answer is b.** She would ignore gibes because they were insulting.

Reading Comprehension

Passage 1

17. **The answer is d.** The Bering Land Bridge is described as connecting Siberia to what is now Alaska. If humans walked across from Siberia, the first ones in North America would have emerged into Alaska.

18. **The answer is a.** According to the passage, you could drive across the bridge, if it still existed, in about an hour. Based on that information, you can infer that the bridge was about as long as a typical mileage per hour, which would put it at choice A, between 50 and 75 miles.

19. **The answer is a.** A land bridge is a piece of land with water on either side that connects two larger pieces of land. That makes it equivalent to an isthmus.

20. **The answer is d.** The author's reason for including this information is to show how the bridge was used to move animals and then human hunters.

21. **The answer is a**. The paragraph primarily puts forth a theory about migration across the land bridge, supporting the theory with discoveries made by ethnologists, from shared religions to similarities in tools and food preservation.

22. **The answer is b**. According to the passage, some Native Americans object to the theory because it challenges their history and status.

Passage 2

23. **The answer is c**. The other choices are either too broad, or are mentioned only briefly or not at all.

24. **The answer is d**. The passage states that sufficient brain development takes place by the early twenties. No other time period is mentioned.

25. **The answer is b**. There is nothing in the passage to support choices a, c, or d.

26. **The answer is a**. None of the procedures mentioned in choices b, c, or d is mentioned in the passage.

27. **The answer is c**. Brain development was the focus of behavior.

28. **The answer is d**. If the amygdalae were larger, more aggressive behavior was recorded. A better-developed brain produces a less hostile teenage boy.

Passage 3

29. **The answer is c**. The main point of this passage is to show how exposure to toxins now can cause health problems later.

30. **The answer is a**. The fact that doctors and researchers are now studying lead exposure might lead to this inference.

31. **The answer is d**. The other choices are contradicted in the passage. Waiting a long time for results would certainly cause difficulty.

32. **The answer is b**. The quote is support for the main ideas of the article.

33. **The answer is c**. The bone is used because lead accumulates there over time.

34. **The answer is a**. Scientists prefer to be able to warn people as quickly as they can. Choices b and c are contradicted by the article, and choice d is irrelevant.

Passage 4

35. **The answer is c**. The article describes how pepper stimulates pigmentation in skin.

36. **The answer is a**. The article clearly states that scientists were studying piperine.

37. **The answer is b**. The cause of pepper's spicy flavor is directly stated in the third paragraph.

38. **The answer is d**. The function of pigmentation is to protect the skin.

39. **The answer is b**. Skin cancer is a serious risk to be avoided under all circumstances.

40. **The answer is d**. Jackson's lack of pigment was not a piperine deficiency (choice a), and steroids are not phototherapy (choice c). Although choice b may be true, it cannot be inferred from this passage. Choice d, on the other hand, is a safe conclusion to draw.

Passage 5

41. **The answer is a**. Scientists are studying the composition of the upper atmosphere—its makeup or structure. None of the other synonyms fits the context in which the word is found.

42. **The answer is c**. It is the size of that surface that the author finds remarkable.

43. **The answer is b**. The three typical courses of study at Arecibo are described in the second paragraph; the exception to these would be choice b.

44. **The answer is d**. To answer this kind of question, simply return to the paragraph in question and think about its main idea. The main idea of the fourth paragraph is established in the initial topic sentence.

45. **The answer is c**. You can often locate an opinion by searching for adjectives or adverbs that are subjective, such as *fascinating* here.

46. **The answer is b**. The remote-control command center will mean that scientists in Texas need not travel to Puerto Rico to use the telescope.

Word Knowledge

47. **The answer is c**. The reasons for giving the awards were considered to be inconsistent and unpredictable.

48. **The answer is b**. *Regurgitate* means to "flow back." A dog can remove poisonous food by vomiting.

49. **The answer is a**. Sixty-two days wandering in a desert would make you look like a dead person, or cadaver.

50. **The answer is b**. A labyrinth is a maze with many walls and hallways.

51. **The answer is b**. The Latin roots of *disparity* combine to mean "inequality."

52. **The answer is a**. To supplant is to take the place of.

53. **The answer is b**. The French word *entourer* means "to surround." An entourage surrounds a star the way planets surround the sun.

54. **The answer is c**. Fallibility can be thought of as the ability to fail.

55. **The answer is a**. Someone who is venerated (as a god might be) is well-respected.

56. **The answer is a**. The ability to assess quickly and accurately requires astuteness, or good judgment.

57. **The answer is c**. Both *deride* and *ridicule* derive from *ridere*, "to laugh."

58. **The answer is a**. A digression is straying off topic while speaking or writing.

59. **The answer is a**. Something that can bend without breaking like a tree limb is supple. The opposite would be something that is not bendable—something rigid.

60. **The answer is c**. A speech to new volunteers would be delivered in easy-to-understand, simple language.

Mathematics

1. **The answer is d**. Align digits by their place values and add.

2. **The answer is c**. The number of donors on Tuesday was about 25, and from Tuesday to Wednesday, that number increased by about 25. That is a 100% increase from Tuesday to Wednesday.

3. **The answer is c**. The decrease from Wednesday to Thursday is the only decrease over 10, which you can tell by estimating using the gridlines on the chart.

4. **The answer is a**. Align digits by their place values and subtract.

5. **The answer is d**. $(23 + 8 + 2 + 7) \div 4 = 10$.

6. **The answer is d**. $\dfrac{7}{35}$ divides out to 0.2.

7. **The answer is c**. To solve this system of equations, begin by:

   (1) $x + y = 4$
   (2) $2x - 6y = 3$

Starting with equation (1), solve for x which results in:

(3) $x = 4 - y$

Substituting equation (3) into equation (2) yields:

(4) $2(4 - y) - 6y = 3$

$8 - 2y - 6y = 3$

$-8y = 3 - 8 = -5$

$8y = 5$

(5) $y = \dfrac{5}{8}$.

Substituting equation (5) into equation (1) yields:

$$x + \left(\frac{5}{8}\right) = 4$$

$$x = 4 - \left(\frac{5}{8}\right) = \frac{32}{8} - \frac{5}{8} = \frac{27}{8}$$

The solutions for the system of equations are $x = \dfrac{27}{8}, y = \dfrac{5}{8}$.

8. **The answer is a.** You should note that $\sqrt[3]{x} = x\frac{1}{3}$ and $x\frac{1}{3} = y^4$. Taking the cube of both sides yields: $\left(x\frac{1}{3}\right)^3 = (y^3)^3$. So $x = y^{12}$.

9. **The answer is a.** The probability of selecting a single orange-colored candy from a bag of Skittles® requires 8 successful outcomes out of 37 possible outcomes. So the probability of selecting a single orange-colored candy is: $p = \dfrac{8}{37}$.

10. **The answer is b.** To determine the probability that a randomly selected card is an ace of a red suit, you should first note that a card can be selected from a deck in $n = 52$ different ways. Since there are two such aces (ace of hearts and ace of diamonds), then an ace can be drawn from the deck in $s = 2$ different ways. Thus, the probability that the selected card is an ace is: $p = \dfrac{s}{n} = \dfrac{2}{52}$.

11. **The answer is b.** The formula for finding the area of a square is $A = s^2$. In this case, the radius of the circle would have to be doubled and then squared: $2 \times 3 \text{ cm}^2 = 6 = 36 \text{ cm}^2$.

12. **The answer is b.** The wall and the floor form the base and height of a right triangle, so the ladder is the hypotenuse. Using the Pythagorean theorem, $a^2 + b^2 = c^2$, plug in the numbers you know and get $8^2 + b^2 = 10^2$. Therefore $b^2 = 36$, and b, the distance on the floor from the wall to the ladder, is 6 feet.

13. **The answer is c.** To find the average, add the numbers and then divide by the number of numerals listed: $(8 + 3 + 6 + 11) \div 4 = 28 \div 4 = 7$.

14. **The answer is c.** Set up a proportion, or two equal fractions, to compare these two scenarios. For example, 6 forms might go in the numerator on the left and 15 minutes in the denominator. Then 30 forms would then go in the numerator on the right, and x or another variable in the denominator. Cross-multiplying gives $6x = 450$, and dividing each side by 6 to solve for x gives 75.

15. **The answer is c.** Be sure to line up the ones, tens, and hundreds columns properly.

16. **The answer is d.** You can translate this statement directly into algebra. The statement "Ryan is 2 years older than four times Pixie's age" becomes $R = 2 + 4P$, which is choice d.

17. **The answer is b.** The longest distance across a circle, which in this case is 10 feet, is the same as its diameter; therefore, the radius is 5 feet. The formula for area of a circle is $A = \pi r$. Thus $A = \pi 5^2$, or 25π.

18. **The answer is a.** The question is asking for the circumference of the tire. Because the radius is 15, you can plug into the formula for circumference and get $C = 2 \times 15 \times \pi$, or 30π.

19. **The answer is d.** Creating two equal fractions for your proportion, you could put 5 (berries) in the numerator and 4 (yogurt) in the denominator on the left, then 10 (yogurt) in the denominator on the right and x in the numerator. Cross-multiplying gives you $50 = 4x$, so $12.5 = x$.

20. **The answer is c.** Simplify to make it easier to translate: J is five more than twice F. Now you can see the mathematical equivalent for each word, $J = 5 + 2F$.

21. **The answer is c.** $33\frac{1}{3}\%$ is the same as $\frac{1}{3}$ of the pie chart. You know that a circle has 360 degrees total, so $\frac{1}{3}$ of 360 is 120 degrees.

22. **The answer is c.** Using the Pythagorean theorem, $4^2 + 6^2 = c^2$. So $52 = c^2$, meaning that $\sqrt{52} = c$. The prime factors of 52 are 2, 2, and 13, so the 2s come outside of the root sign and $2\sqrt{13}$ is the result.

23. **The answer is b.** The prime factors of 80 are 2, 2, 2, 2, and 5, so the two pairs of 2s can come outside of the square root sign and the 5 must stay in.

24. **The answer is a.** Set up a proportion between similar triangles and corresponding sides. With like sides as a ratio: $\frac{2}{4} = \frac{6}{x}$. $2x = 24; x = 12$.

25. **The answer is d.** Be sure to set up a proportion: 2 walls and 90 minutes are on the left and 6 walls and x are on the right. Cross-multiplying gives $2x = 540$. Divide both sides by 2 and you have $x = 270$.

26. **The answer is a.** $1.77 \times 3 = 5.31$ so $\dfrac{5.31}{3} = 1.77$. When dividing, align the decimal point in the quotient with the decimal point in the dividend.

27. **The answer is c.** When solving a multiplication problem like this one, take care when carrying numbers over.

28. **The answer is b.** Once you pare down the excess words, the problem is really asking what is 20% of 35, which is also $\dfrac{1}{5}$ of 35. $\dfrac{1}{5} \times 35 = 7$.

29. **The answer is c.** First, you need to reduce. The fraction $\dfrac{60}{40}$ reduces to $2\dfrac{1}{2}$ or 2.5. Expressed as a percentage, $2.5 = 250\%$.

30. **The answer is b.** This is a basic proportion problem; set up 5 over 2 on one side and 30 over x on the other side. Cross-multiply and you get $5x = 60$, which solves to $x = 12$.

31. **The answer is d.** You can eliminate choice a and b with one multiplication and c with two.

32. **The answer is a.** By locating Mr. Smith's temperature on the chart at the start and the end of each hour, the amount of change can be determined. It changed about 2.1° during hours 1 and 2 (from about 99.2° to about 101.3°). It changed about 1.9° during hours 3 and 4 (from 100.5° to about 98.6°).

33. **The answer is d.** This problem is basic translation, but be careful about the meaning of "three years younger"; it can be tricky to tell when you need to subtract.

34. **The answer is b.** Let's translate: "5 is what percent of 40" becomes $5 = \dfrac{x}{100} \times 40$, or $5 = \dfrac{40x}{100}$. Multiply both sides by 100 and you get $500 = 40x$; divide each side by 40 and you get $12.5 = x$. Therefore, 5 is 12.5% of 40.

35. **The answer is a.** Double 46 to realize the answer has to start with 1.

36. **The answer is d.** The number of total possible outcomes from the roll of two dice is 36. In other words, there are 36 different pairs of numbers that can be obtained. You first need to determine the number of possible outcomes yielding a sum of 7 and 12 from the two dice.

The number of possible outcomes yielding a sum of 7 is 6 or $\{(1, 6), (2, 5), (3, 4), (4, 3), (5, 2), (6, 1)\}$.

The probability of yielding a sum of 7 between the two dice is

$$P(A) = P(7) = \frac{6}{36} = \frac{1}{6}.$$

The number of possible outcomes yielding a sum of 12 is 1 or

$\{(6,6)\}$.

The probability of yielding a sum of 12 between the two dice is

$$P(B) = P(12) = \frac{1}{36}.$$

Upon the roll of two dice, you cannot obtain a sum of 7 and a sum of 12 at the same time; thus, the two outcomes are mutually exclusive. The probability that the sum of the two dice is either 7 or 12 is: $P(A \text{ or } B) = P(A) + (B) = P(7) + P(12) = 6/36 + 1/36 = 7/36$.

37. **The answer is b.** Because the two drawings are made from a complete deck of cards, the two events are independent of one another. You first need to determine the probability of drawing a card of two suits from a deck of cards. Out of a total of 52 cards, there are 13 cards of any suit and 26 cards of a black suit. The probability of drawing a card of a black suit, $P(A)$, is $\frac{26}{52}$. Because the first card is replaced before the second drawing, the probability of drawing a card of the same suit, $P(B)$, is also $\frac{26}{52}$. Thus, the probability of drawing two cards of the same suit is $P(A \text{ and } B) = P(A) \cdot P(B) = \frac{26}{52} \cdot \frac{26}{52} = \frac{676}{2,704}$.

38. **The answer is c.** The mean of a data set is the arithmetic average of the values of the data set or

$$\frac{2.4\,\text{mL} + 3.2\,\text{mL} + 3.7\,\text{mL} + 3.7\,\text{mL} + 4.5\,\text{mL} + 6.8\,\text{mL} + 7.3\,\text{mL} + 8.1\,\text{mL} + 12.2\,\text{mL}}{9}$$

$$= \frac{51.9\,\text{mL}}{9} \cong 5.8\,\text{mL}$$

39. **The answer is b.** The median is the middle or center value of the data set arranged in ascending numerical order, or 4.5 mL.

40. **The answer is a.** The mode is the measurement that is the most frequent or common value in the data set. In this example, the mode is 3.7 mL, because it occurs twice, more than any of the other measurements that occur only once.

Science

1. **The answer is d.** Acceleration is defined as the change in velocity over time, $a = \frac{\Delta v}{\Delta t}$.

2. **The answer is b.** Momentum, p, is equal to mass times velocity. Choice b has the least momentum, 20 kg·m/s.

3. **The answer is b.** The equation for momentum reflects mass multiplied by velocity.

4. **The answer is c.** Because the equation for momentum multiplies mass (kg) and velocity (m/s), the units are kg·m/s.

5. **The answer is d.** The Newton is the unit of measure for force, which is calculated by the formula $F = ma$. Multiplying mass (kg) by acceleration (m/s^2) gives kg·m/s^2.

6. **The answer is a.** Enzymes break down proteins and pepsin in a variety of forms in the stomach. Mucus protects the stomach lining, hormones stimulate acids, and ions join to create hydrochloric acid to break down foods.

7. **The answer is c.** These other vessels are veins or parts of the heart.

8. **The answer is c.** A photon is an energy packet of electromagnetic radiation in the visible range. An electron and a neutrino are names for much larger elementary particles like the muon.

9. **The answer is d.** Ohm's law states that resistance is voltage divided by current.

10. **The answer is b.** Smooth muscles make up most of the internal organs.

11. **The answer is a.** Striations or bands are found in cardiac and skeletal muscles but not in smooth muscle. Cardiac and smooth muscle cells have a single nucleus, while skeletal muscles have core elements called nuclei.

12. **The answer is d.** By tracing the increase in volume along the x-axis, a corresponding rise in the y-axis can be measured along the same ratio line.

13. **The answer is b.** The density of a medium determines how fast sound passes through it. Iron is the most dense of any of these materials and sound moves through it at 5,130 m/s at 20°C. Glass is close to iron's density and sound would pass at 4,540 m/s. Wood would be next at 3,850 m/s and water would be last at 1,500 m/s.

14. **The answer is c.** Plasma is a mixture of elections and positively charged ions. It exists only in lightening bolts or in stars where temperatures are high enough to created it. Crystals are the lattice structure of ions formed through evaporation or cooling iconic solids. Atoms that take on or give up electrons are ions but this is not a fourth state of matter to go with the other three, solid, liquid, and gas. Zeolites are ion-exchange resins made up of mineral substances.

15. **The answer is b.** Objects can be classified by how their material reacts to light. A glass brick is made up of very thick glass, which allows some light to come through but you can't really see any details through it. Something like glass allows almost all the light that strikes it to pass through reflecting only a small portion of

light. Reflective is a substance that redirects some or all of the light hitting it. A substance is opaque if it absorbs or reflects light striking it.

16. **The answer is d.** Interior tissues and bone in the human body can be scanned without an operation though the use of rays that penetrate different matter in different ways. These rays are then used to form images. MRI stands for magnetic resonance imaging. Powerful magnets excite hydrogen nuclei in water molecules within the body, which give off a detectable signal. Radiography uses X-rays. CT also uses X-rays but instead of one beam as in traditional X-rays, a CT scan uses hundreds of beams in an arc, forming a far more detailed image. Ultrasound uses sound waves as they pass through different structures to reveal details.

17. **The answer is c.** Bones provide structure for the human body which would otherwise collapse of its own weight and softness without them. However, muscles, not bones, actually provide movement by flexing or extending which moves the bones to which they are attached. Bones form a cage around internal organs, providing protection. The marrow inside bones supplies the body with blood cells. The hardness of bones comes from minerals, one of which, calcium, can be absorbed or broken down as needed by a process called resorption.

18. **The answer is d.** If a car travels 3 miles north, 6 miles south, 2 miles east, 2 miles west, and then 3 miles north, it has traveled a total distance of 16 miles. But because of the directions the car has traveled in, it has ended up in the same place from which it started. This means that the displacement of the car is zero.

19. **The answer is a.** Using the equation $a = \Delta \dfrac{v}{t}$, the car has a final velocity of 0 m/s and an initial velocity of 5 m/s. The change in velocity is –5 m/s. Dividing this by the time, 2.5 seconds, the acceleration is –2 m/s².

20. **The answer is a.** The velocity of the car is equal to the time multiplied by the acceleration. Multiplying 5 seconds by 10 m/s², you get a velocity of 50 m/s.

21. **The answer is a.** Momentum is calculated by multiplying mass and velocity, $p = mv$. Although the meteorite sounds intimidating, it is the car that has the greatest momentum at 6,250 kg • m/s.

22. **The answer is c.** Applying Newton's second law, $F = ma$, a 1.0-kg block accelerated at 6 m/s² requires a 6-N force to move it.

23. **The answer is d.** Work is the force that is applied to an object over a distance, $W = Fd$. The force is 15 N and distance is 3 m, giving a total amount of work equal to 45 N • m.

24. **The answer is d.** The equation of the velocity of a wave is $v = f\lambda$. This is the multiplication of frequency by wavelength.

25. **The answer is a.** The correct unit for current is amperes.

26. **The answer is b.** The symbol shown is the symbol for ohms, the unit for resistance.

27. **The answer is d.** Rearranging the equation, we find that the current is equal to the voltage divided by the resistance, $I = \dfrac{V}{R}$.

28. **The answer is a.** Lights connected in parallel have an advantage over those connected in series in that, should one lightbulb break or burn out, the others will remain lit.

29. **The answer is b.** The voltage, V, is equal to IR, current times resistance.

30. **The answer is d.** Electrical potential is measured in volts. The other three choices, ohms, watts, and amperes are resistance, power, and current, respectively.

31. **The answer is a.** Newton's first law addresses inertia and states that an object at rest will stay at rest and that an object in motion will stay in motion. This changes if the object is acted on by a force.

32. **The answer is b.** Acceleration of an object requires a force. This can be calculated using the equation $F = ma$, as described by Newton's second law.

33. **The answer is c.** Newton's third law states that when an object applies a force to a second object, that second object applies an opposite and equal force to the first object.

34. **The answer is c.** For the object to come to rest, a force must act on it. One possible force is the friction that exists between the object and the table.

35. **The answer is c.** Work, W, is equal to force times distance, Fd. This gives, using the correct units, 15 N·m.

36. **The answer is b.** $W = Fd$ or $F = \dfrac{W}{d}$. The work, 100 N·m, divided by 20 meters, gives a force of 5 N.

37. **The answer is a.** Conservation of energy tells us that energy can neither be created nor destroyed. The total energy of a system, however, can be converted from one form to another.

38. **The answer is d.** Energy is measured in joules. Height is a distance, d, and is measured in meters.

39. **The answer is a.** The term *olfactory* refers to the nose and nasal cavity.

40. **The answer is d.** The noble gases are located in the rightmost group/family on the periodic table. They are very stable atoms because they have a full octet of valence electrons.

41. **The answer is a.** When light or any energy passes through a medium, it is affected by the properties of that medium. A higher refractive index makes for a greater. Air has a refractive index of 1.00 and has little effect on yellow light.

42. **The answer is a.** Choices b and d would involve experimentation. Choice c will only give information about expressed traits. Certain diseases can be traced through inheritance patterns in a family tree or a pedigree chart.

43. **The answer is d.** The pairings for DNA are guanine with cytosine and thymine with adenine. Uracil is found in RNA, where it pairs with adenine.

44. **The answer is c.** Nucleic acids make up DNA, which codes for how humans develop.

45. **The answer is b.** Red blood cells contain hemoglobin, which is responsible for transporting oxygen throughout the body.

46. **The answer is a.** The cell membrane is said to be selectively permeable, controlling what enters and exits the cell.

47. **The answer is d.** Meiosis describes cell divisions and results with each cell having two chromosomes. In Mitosis, each cell ends up having two pairs of chromosomes identical to the parent cell. Both begin with two chromatids but only in mitosis do homologous chromosome spindle individually and identical sets move in opposite directions.

48. **The answer is a.** Rod cells distinguish black and white. At dusk or even in near darkness they allow us to see shapes. Cone cells detect colors. The lens focuses light as it comes through a single cornea, which controls the flow of light into the eye. The optic nerve conveys sensations to the brain.

49. **The answer is c.** As the diver stands on the cliff, she has maximum potential energy. As she starts her fall, her gravitational potential energy is highest as gravity acts on her body falling and she starts to build up some kinetic energy. As she hits the water, gravitational potential energy is gone and maximum kinetic energy occurs. When she stops falling and surfaces, she has no more kinetic energy or gravitational potential energy.

50. **The answer is d.** If a negatively charged object is brought near a positively-charged object, the electrons that are positively charged are repelled and move away. If direct contact were to be made, conduction would occur and positively charged electrons would flow from one object to the other. In friction, contact between two objects removes electrons from the surface of one object, which then attach to the other object. Insulation prevents any electrical charges from flowing between two objects.

51. **The answer is a.** Diabetics have difficulty controlling blood-sugar levels in their kidneys. Their blood-sugar levels are too high and they excrete blood-sugar as glucose into their urine. A low-blood sugar condition is caused by too much insulin or other diseases and can be dangerous.

52. **The answer is d.** Sunlight is made up of different wavelengths which produce the different colors of the spectrum. Due to the curvature of the Earth, sunlight at dusk has to pass through more air due to its low angle and other colors are blocked, leaving red or yellow to dominate. At noon, the higher angle of the sun in the sky means it passes through less air so the blue wavelength dominates. When the sky is blue on one place on Earth, it can be red or other colors somewhere else. Dust in the air during the day could block sunlight but would have to exist in high concentrations to block out blue.

53. **The answer is b.** *Reflection* takes place when light bounces back at the same angle at which it hits an object. *Refraction* takes place when light changes speed as it goes from one medium to another. *Diffraction* is the bending of waves around obstacles in their path.

54. **The answer is a.** Using the equation $V = IR$ or $R = \dfrac{V}{I}$, an electronic device connected to a 6-volt source drawing 3 amperes has a total resistance of 2 ohms.

55. **The answer is b.** Force is equal to mass times acceleration ($F = ma$). This is the equation for Newton's second law.

56. **The answer is c.** Refraction is the bending of light that takes place as light travels from one medium into another. It occurs because of the change in speed of the light.

57. **The answer is a.** Power can be found by multiplying V by I. This gives 220 watts of power.

58. **The answer is d.** According to the equation $P = IV$, the current is $\dfrac{P}{V}$. Dividing 1,525 watts by 110 volts gives 13.9 amperes.

59. **The answer is a.** Only choice a demonstrates the correct units for impulse, N·s. In addition, the impulse can be calculated by multiplying the force by the change in time, $p = F\Delta t$.

60. **The answer is d.** The 10-kg object had a change in its velocity by 10 m/s. Using the equation $p = m\Delta v$, we find that the correct answer is 100 kg·m/s.

Practice Test 4

Verbal Ability Word Knowledge

1. **The answer is b.** When someone is very comfortable, they are lazy and relaxed, or indolent.

2. **The answer is c.** In ancient times, a harbinger was an advance man from an army or royal entourage.

3. **The answer is a**. The surgeon is a favorite, so she would be praising his or her virtues.

4. **The answer is c**. If you endeavor to do something, you make an effort to do it.

5. **The answer is b**. At a funeral, a speech in praise of the deceased is a eulogy.

6. **The answer is c**. The sun's apex or its highest point in the sky is also called a zenith.

7. **The answer is c**. An area that is rubbed or activated into a response is stimulated.

8. **The answer is b**. *Severe* has multiple meanings. One of them is *austere*, or *stern*.

9. **The answer is c**. Literally, an aversion is a turning away. It is used to describe a feeling of intense dislike.

10. **The answer is d**. A domineering official would assert authority in a bossy, or officious, manner.

11. **The answer is b**. To satiate is to fill up, or satisfy.

12. **The answer is c**. Someone who is sanguine has a sunny outlook on life.

13. **The answer is a**. To delve is to dig into, either literally or figuratively, as when one delves into one's past.

14. **The answer is a**. Someone who is impudent or audacious would have the nerve to confront a chef.

15. **The answer is a**. To foment in medicine is to apply a poultice or treat with warm water. To foment in other contexts is to stimulate.

16. **The answer is a**. Substitute each word in the sentence and see which one works.

Reading Comprehension

Passage 1

17. **The answer is c**. The fifth paragraph says that it is "impervious to burning."

18. **The answer is a**. The entire passage deals with a floral invader.

19. **The answer is c**. In the second paragraph: "The same long growing season that makes it so beloved by gardeners makes it a seed-making machine." It is the long growing season that gardeners like.

20. **The answer is d**. Although *dense* has a variety of meanings, here the author is referring to the thickness of the stands, not their opacity or complexity. The weeds are tightly concentrated.

21. **The answer is d.** Because loosestrife thrives in wetlands and along rivers, the places it would **most** easily thrive include swamps, wetland meadows, and along inland waterways.

22. **The answer is b.** If a new strain of purple loosestrife is growing up where it was once eliminated, then this form of eradication does not really work.

Passage 2

23. **The answer is b.** The statement about naps is based on the facts in the passage.

24. **The answer is d.** Appetite was not mentioned in the passage.

25. **The answer is c.** The improvement of a person's memory is mentioned in the passage as a side effect.

26. **The answer is a.** Only allowing a person mentally to sort out important and unnecessary information was actually named as a purpose of sleep.

27. **The answer is d.** The effectiveness of catnaps is the basic conclusion of the passage.

28. **The answer is a.** When sorting temporary information into permanent storage or discarding it, the brain frees up space for more information and more learning.

Passage 3

29. **The answer is b.** This title best summarizes the thrust of the article by focusing on the pyramid's changes.

30. **The answer is a.** Getting older people to change their eating habits is the overall idea of the article.

31. **The answer is c.** Only drinking adequate fluids is actually associated with helping proper digestion.

32. **The answer is d.** The fact that they have a much longer shelf life is the reason dried and frozen fruits are recommended.

33. **The answer is c.** The author is deliberately suggesting forms of exercise that would not be risky for older adults.

34. **The answer is a.** The purpose of the passage is to alert readers to the different dietary needs of seniors.

Passage 4

35. **The answer is d.** The article provides basic information about the condition itself and the sources of folic acid.

36. **The answer is b.** According to the article, women should be sure to have enough folic acid even before they conceive.

37. **The answer is c.** Rereading the final sentence should indicate that folic acid can lower the risk (without preventing it entirely) of a number of diseases.

38. **The answer is d.** The last paragraph indicates that folic acid helps prevent breast cancer, among other conditions, but that does not mean that breast cancer is caused by a lack of folic acid.

39. **The answer is b.** Only the word *tarnishes* could be substituted into the sentence where *mars* is used.

40. **The answer is a.** A topical shot is never mentioned as an option, so choice a is the correct answer.

Passage 5

41. **The answer is b.** The author uses the word *incredibly* to describe the fact that nearly every ape on the planet appears on the Red List. Her tone is that of someone who is shocked at this information.

42. **The answer is b.** According to the third paragraph, in areas with Ebola, it wipes out 90% of the gorillas. That leaves 1 in 10.

43. **The answer is c.** The only way to answer this question is to refer back to the sentences indicated. Here they are: (1) "The Western Lowland gorilla moved from 'endangered' to 'critically endangered' in 2007." (2) " 'Critically endangered' indicates that its population and range are shrinking, and it is in imminent danger of extinction." Sentence 2 defines the term *critically endangered* that is used in sentence 1.

44. **The answer is c.** Every part of the passage indicates that human behavior is harming the great apes in general and gorillas in particular.

45. **The answer is a.** The author begins the fifth paragraph with the statement: "The number one threat to gorillas, however, is human greed." She then supports this hypothesis with examples.

46. **The answer is d.** The author ends with the grim assessment: "Some give these vegetarian cousins of *Homo sapiens* no more than a decade before all wild specimens are eradicated."

Word Knowledge

47. **The answer is c.** The key words are *yesterday's* and *typewriters*, which hint at the past. The prefix *ante-* means *before* and *deluvian* refers to a flood (deluge), so the word itself refers to a time before Noah's flood, or ancient times.

48.   **The answer is a.** *Squalor* refers to filth or complete uncleanliness.

49.   **The answer is a.** An older, more experienced colleague would tutor someone as a mentor, or guide.

50.   **The answer is b.** Relationships between governments are governed by protocol, or codes of behavior and action.

51.   **The answer is c.** In essence, the meaning of *paraphrase* is "to speak similarly," or to use one's own words to restate someone else's.

52.   **The answer is c.** *Tacit* means "unspoken" or "silent." Someone who is taciturn is certainly not outgoing.

53.   **The answer is d.** A doctor would not want to volunteer information that would upset a patient.

54.   **The answer is a.** To soothe or calm an anxious patient, a doctor might sedate him or her.

55.   **The answer is d.** A testimonial testifies to someone's good deeds or character.

56.   **The answer is a.** In Latin, *corpus* means body, so having plenty of body is being overweight.

57.   **The answer is a.** To tell the difference is to discriminate or distinguish between choices.

58.   **The answer is d.** Rather than one constant achievement, Kevin had a series of intermittent, or sporadic ones.

59.   **The answer is b.** To shudder is to move back and forth, and turbulent motion is also back and forth.

60.   **The answer is c.** Someone with hypochondria has abnormal anxiety about his or her health.

Mathematics

1.   **The answer is c.** The fraction $\frac{8}{2}$ reduces to 4. To convert to a percent, just move the decimal two places to the right, which gives 400%.

2.   **The answer is d.** Multiplying 287 by 10 would be 2,870 or nearly 3,000, so multiplying 287 by 36 has to produce an answer closer to 10,000 than 9,000 something.

3.   **The answer is c.** Because prime numbers are divisible only by themselves and 1, the even numbers—36 and 38—are not prime. The number 35 is also divisible by 5 and 7, so it cannot be prime. The number 37 is the only answer choice that fits.

4. **The answer is d.** When you solve for x, you get:

$$3 - 3 + 4x = 23 - 3$$
$$4x = 20$$
$$\frac{4x}{4} = \frac{20}{4}$$
$$x = 5.$$

5. **The answer is c.** First, you need to convert the mixed number, $1\frac{2}{3}$, to an improper fraction. Multiplying the integer by the denominator, you get 3, which you then add to the numerator to get $\frac{5}{3}$. Using the bowtie method to add $\frac{5}{3}$ and $\frac{4}{5}$ gives $\frac{25}{15} + \frac{12}{15}$, which equals $\frac{37}{15}$.

6. **The answer is d.** Answering this question is mainly about making sure you are looking up the correct information in the table. The 2001 Bordeaux has the highest sales in cases, which is really all the information you need.

7. **The answer is b.** To find what percentage of sales was in individual bottles, just consider the number of individual bottles divided by the number of bottles total. Because the math on this one is pretty time-consuming, "ballpark" first to see if you can eliminate any answer choices. For the 1997 Pinot Noir, approximately 15,000 divided by approximately 80,000 is a little less than 20%. For the 1994 Pinot Gris, approximately 18,000 divided by approximately 77,000 is about 23%, or almost 25%. For the 1991 Chardonnay, approximately 15,000 divided by approximately 90,000 is about 20%. For the 2001 Bordeaux, approximately 12,000 divided by approximately 100,000 is about 12%. So the 1994 Pinot Gris has definitely the largest percentage of sales in individual bottles.

8. **The answer is a.** Subtracting 3 from 7 should leave 4, but the hundreds digits force you to borrow, so it has to be 3.

9. **The answer is c.** Remember, when you see a division sign and the bases are the same, you can just subtract the exponents.

10. **The answer is c.** Because the only difference between the answer choices in this problem is the number of places behind the decimal, all you really need to do is count. There are three places behind the decimal in the original problem; therefore, there are three places behind the decimal in the result.

11. **The correct choice is b.** 0.6×70, or $6 \times 70 = 420$ and then you move the decimal one place to the left, giving you 42.

12. **The correct choice is b.** You can use the Pythagorean theorem on this problem, but it is also a Pythagorean shortcut. A triangle with sides 30, 40, and 50 is similar to a triangle with sides 3, 4, and 5.

13. **The correct choice is d.** Cherry pie has 29%, so you need to find other categories that add up to 29. Blueberry, peach, and key lime have 29%, collectively, so choice d is the correct answer.

14. **The correct choice is d.** You are looking for an answer choice (or two) that would give you greater than 42%, collectively. Clearly choice b is greater than 42%, because it encompasses all the categories except apple and, therefore, totals 58%. Peach, key lime, and cherry add up to 50%, so choice c also works, making choice d the correct answer.

15. **The answer is d.** This question is mostly a basic proportion, with 45 minutes over 1 day on the left and x over 7 days (remember to convert!) on the right. Cross-multiply and you get $315 = x$. However, the answer choices are expressed in hours *and* minutes, so you must divide 315 by 60 (the number of minutes in one hour) to get 5 r15, or 5 hours, 15 minutes.

16. **The answer is d.** Because 1 inch equals approximately 2.5 centimeters, multiply 48 by 2.5. Even if you only ballpark, 120 is the only answer that comes close.

17. **The answer is d.** Because the problem is looking for area of a rectangular field, you just need to add the portions of the length and the width to get totals, then multiply the length and the width. $(45 + 45) \times (42 + 43) = 90 \times 85 = 7,650$.

18. **The answer is d.** First, convert the integer and mixed number into improper fractions. 3 becomes $\dfrac{3}{1}$ and $1\dfrac{5}{6}$ becomes $\dfrac{11}{6}$. You can bowtie $\dfrac{3}{1} - \dfrac{11}{6}$ to equal $\dfrac{18}{6} - \dfrac{11}{6}$, which becomes $\dfrac{7}{6}$.

19. **The answer is c.** Remember to factor the 2 out of both terms; there is an answer choice that is otherwise correct, and it does not have the 2. Otherwise, the greatest number of x's that you can factor out is 4, and the greatest number of y's you can factor out is 3; the part inside the parentheses remains the same in all answer choices, so you do not even need to worry about the rest.

20. **The answer is a.** Translate: "Bob is 5,000 less than the sum of Al and Carl" (yes, the problem is actually talking about their salaries, but we are simplifying the language) translates to $B = -5,000 + A + C$, which can be rearranged to fit choice a.

21. **The answer is d.** The range, or the difference between the largest and smallest values in this data set, is 12.2 mL – 2.4 mL = 9.8 mL.

22. **The answer is d.** The first thing to do in solving the equation $x^2 - 12x = -36$ for x is to rewrite the equation by adding 36 to both sides and then to express the equation in terms of factors:

$x^2 - 12x + 36 = 0$
$(x - 6) \cdot (x - 6) = 0$
Solving the equation for x yields $x = 6$.

23. **The answer is a.** Divide each term by x to get a difference of squares, $x^2 - 64$, on the left side and 0 on the right side. Then factor.

24. **The answer is c.** This equation can be solved by first taking the square root of both sides of the equation

$$\sqrt{(4x-1)^2} = \sqrt{121}$$
$$4x - 1 = 11$$

Solving for x yields $x = 3$.

25. **The answer is d.** Use the formula to convert to Fahrenheit.

26. **The answer is b.** To convert from Fahrenheit to Celsius, subtract 32 and multiply by $\frac{5}{9}$. The calculation $(90 - 32) \times \frac{5}{9} = 58 \times \frac{5}{9}$ gives a little more than half of 58. Choice b is the only one that is close.

27. **The answer is c.** If the length and width of the room are the same (and are integers, which they must be according to the answer choices), then a good knowledge of square roots helps solve the problem. The number 14 squared is 196, so 14 is the length and width of the room.

28. **The answer is b.** Ignoring the decimals, $398 \times 72 = 28,656$. There are four spaces to the right of the decimal (collectively) in 3.98 and 0.72, so move the decimal four spaces to the left and get 2.8656.

29. **The answer is c.** Constructing a proportion, or two equal fractions, is again a good way to go. The fraction on the left has 3 in the numerator and 2 in the denominator, and the fraction on the right has 9 in the numerator and x in the denominator. Cross-multiply and get $3x = 9 \times 2$, and solve to get $3x = 18$, or $x = 6$.

30. **The answer is c.** The prime factors of 30 are 2, 3, and 5, and their sum is 10.

31. **The answer is c.** $(8 + -4 + 3 + 9 + 4) \div 5 = 4$.

32. **The answer is c.** First, you must convert the mixed number into an improper fraction. $2 \times 4 + 3 = 11$, so you get $\frac{11}{4}$ for our improper fraction. Second, dividing by a fraction means you need to flip it and multiply, so your problem is really $\frac{11}{8} \times \frac{8}{7}$. Multiply across and you get $\frac{88}{28}$, which reduces to $\frac{22}{7}$.

33. **The answer is d.** The formula for the area of a circle is $A = \pi r$, so when you divide the circumference of 12 by 2 and then plug in a radius of 6 and get $A = \pi 6^2$, the area is 36π.

34. **The answer is c.** 15 and 1 should be 16, but look to the hundreds digits, which will total more than 10.

35. **The answer is a**. First, look at the easiest thing to tell at first glance; the line crosses the y-axis at 1, so you can eliminate choices b and a. The slope is $\frac{1}{3}$, which you distinguish from 3 by ballparking, because it is a very gradual slope, or you can determine it using *rise/run*.

36. **The answer is a**. The quotient of the two fractions can be found by writing the fractions as: $\frac{1}{3} \div \frac{5}{9} = \left(\frac{1}{3}\right) " \left(\frac{9}{5}\right) = \frac{3}{5}$.

37. **The answer is d**. The average of a set of numbers is calculated by:

$$= \frac{24+53+70+89+34+30}{6} = \frac{300}{6} = 50$$

38. **The answer is c**. The number 239 is expressed in scientific notation by first expressing the value in terms of a real number such that $1 \le a < 10$. In this case, the number becomes 2.39. In order to retain the original number, the number must be multiplied by 100 which, in terms of exponents, is 10^2. Thus, in scientific notation, $239 = 2.39 \times 100 = 2.39 \times 10^2$.

39. **The answer is b**. To divide the two numbers in scientific notation, you have:

$$-5.4 \times 10^7 \div 2.7 \times 10^3 = -5.4 \times \frac{10^7}{2.7} \times 10^3 = -\frac{5.4}{2.7} \times \frac{10^7}{10^3} = -2.0 \times 10^4$$

40. **The answer is c**. To solve the inequality $3x - 9 > 1 - 2x$, you need to collect like terms of x on one side of the inequality and all other values to the other side. You first add 9 to both sides of the inequality:

$3x - 9 + 9 > 1 - 2x + 9$
$3x > 10 - 2x$.

You then add $2x$ to both sides of the inequality:

$3x + 2x > 10 - 2x + 2x$
$5x > 10$.

Dividing both sides by 5 yields $x > 2$.

Science

1. **The answer is c**. Because plants need light to survive, they tend to bend toward light sources. This tendency is termed *phototropism*.

2. **The answer is d**. Changes in the base sequences in DNA can lead to the coding of different proteins. These mutations can eventually lead to cancer.

3. **The answer is c.** Tinctures are solutions in which the solute is dissolved into alcohol.

4. **The answer is d.** The gain or loss of electrons is what causes ions to form. Positive ions form because atoms have lost a negatively charged electron.

5. **The answer is c.** Fifty percent of the plants will be tall because, as a Punnett square would show, two of the new allele sets will be Tt and the other two will be tt.

6. **The answer is d.** If a Punnett square is created showing the cross between a color-blind male (X'Y') and a female carrier (X'X), the resulting combinations will be X'X, X'Y, X'X, and XY. The underline offspring are color-blind.

	X'	**Y**
X'	X'X' Color-blind female	X'Y Color-blind male
X	X'X	XY

7. **The answer is a.** Mutualism is a relationship in which two organisms live symbiotically and both benefit.

8. **The answer is c.** The burning of fossil fuels has raised levels of carbon dioxide, a greenhouse gas, in the atmosphere. This is believed to be the cause of global warming.

9. **The answer is b.** This example shows a food chain because only one pathway of energy transfer has been diagramed. A food web would show multiple pathways by which the energy from an organism could be passed along.

10. **The answer is b.** A negative velocity indicates that an object is slowing down. If the airplane were at a constant speed, the rate of change would be zero.

11. **The answer is d.** Distance is speed multiplied by time, $d = vt$. Multiplying 4 meters per second by 20 seconds gives 80 meters.

12. **The answer is a.** Isotopes have the same number of protons and are the same element. What makes them different is the number of neutrons present, which makes the mass number vary as well.

13. **The answer is a.** *Amphi* means both (amphitheater, amphibian). An amphoteric substance can act as either an acid or a base.

14. **The answer is c.** In a chemical reaction, a compound may be broken down and transformed into other compounds. Elements, however, are not broken down chemically during a reaction.

15. **The answer is d.** A hydronium ion concentration of 1×10^{-7} M in a solution translates into the solution having a pH of 7. This pH value indicates a neutral solution that is neither acidic nor basic.

16.   **The answer is c.** After 24 days, the sample has undergone three half-lives. During the three half-lives, we see that the amounts change as follows: 1 whole → $\frac{1}{2}$ → $\frac{1}{4}$ → $\frac{1}{8}$, where an arrow represents eight days (one half-life).

17.   **The answer is d.** The plane traveled a total distance of 1,000 miles, but because the plane returned to its original point of origin, its displacement is 0 miles.

18.   **The answer is c.** The reaction $2NaI + Cl_2 → 2NaCl + I_2$ shows a single replacement as the chlorine replaces just one element, the iodine.

19.   **The answer is c.** When attached to the electromagnet, the potential energy (*PE*) of the car is 367.5 kJ because $PE = mgh$, and $PE = (1,500 \text{ kg})(9.8 \text{ m/s}^2)(25 \text{ m})$. As the car falls, all 367.5 kJ of potential energy are converted to kinetic energy. On hitting the ground and making a sound, the car will no longer possess any potential energy.

20.   **The answer is d.** The valence electrons are the outermost electrons in an atom. These electrons are of importance because they are the electrons that are lost, gained, or shared in a reaction.

21.   **The answer is b.** Litmus, red or blue, is blue in a base and red in an acid. Phenolphthalein is colorless in acid and pink in base.

22.   **The answer is d.** The alcohol functional group is the group that has an −OH group bonded to the carbon chain. The other choices show an ether, an alkyne, and an aldehyde, respectively.

23.   **The answer is d.** Values for pH just above 7 are basic. Given that the pH of this blood is just above 7, it indicates that the blood sample is a weak base.

24.   **The answer is c.** Sulfur is located on the upper-right side of the periodic table. It is soft, lacks luster, and does not conduct heat or electricity, making it a nonmetal.

25.   **The answer is d.** Isomers are organic compounds with the same molecular formulas but different structures. Examples are CH_3CH_2OH (an alcohol) and CH_3OCH_3 (an ether). Do not confuse isomers with isotopes, which have the same number of protons and are the same element. What makes isotopes different is the number of neutrons present, which makes the mass number vary as well.

26.   **The answer is b.** See the following diagram:

6 grams → (20 years) →3 grams → (20 years, 40 years total) → 1.5 grams

After 20 years, the 6 grams you started out with will be 3 grams. After another 20 years (40 years total), one-half of 3 grams (1.5 grams) will remain.

27.   **The answer is b.** Zygotes settle in the uterus and develop into embryos.

28.   **The answer is d.** The placenta develops to "connect" the mother to the fetus so that the fetus can obtain oxygen and nutrients.

29. **The answer is a**. Villi, like root tips, are designed to increase the surface area in which absorption occurs.

30. **The answer is d**. *Biomes* are large regions inhabited by ecologically similar communities of living organisms. Examples are deserts, the tundra, and tropical rainforests. A city neighborhood is not a biome.

31. **The answer is d**. The scientific name of an organism reflects its genus and species.

32. **The answer is a**. Finding the exact age of a fossil by examining a rock layer is impossible. A rock layer can, however, give an approximate age of a fossil.

33. **The answer is b**. The idea that all organisms have a fair and equal chance of surviving is not the case. Organisms must compete for survival and resources. Only those that survive can pass on their genes to offspring, and those genes will produce physical characteristics that aid survival.

34. **The answer is d**. Carbon-12 is not an emanation of a nuclear decay. Radioactive substances that undergo a natural transmutation give off alpha particles, beta particles, and gamma rays.

35. **The answer is d**. A strong acid has a very low pH value and more hydronium ions present in solution.

36. **The answer is a**. The symbol for potassium is K (for calcium, Ca; for carbon, C; and for phosphorus, P).

37. **The answer is d**. Exothermic reactions release heat, whereas endothermic reactions absorb heat.

38. **The answer is b**. Boyle's law demonstrates the inversely proportional relationship between pressure and volume. This should not be confused with Charles' law, which relates temperature to volume.

39. **The answer is c**. An ionic bond is formed between a metal and a nonmetal. The metal (Mg) loses electrons to the nonmetal (Br).

40. **The answer is a**. The ability to evaporate is a liquid's volatility. A more volatile liquid evaporates faster.

41. **The answer is a**. Nonpolar compounds have no overall polarity. Diatomic molecules, such as F_2, have two of the same element chemically bonded. Because the elements have the same electronegativity, they share the electrons equally and form a nonpolar covalent bond.

42. **The answer is c**. Sublimation is a change from solid phase to gas phase with no liquid phase in between. Other substances that can sublime are dry ice (solid carbon dioxide) and mothballs (naphthalene).

43.   **The answer is b.** The upper-right portion of the periodic table includes the non-metals. These include the noble gases, halogens, and the elements S, P, O, N, and C.

44.   **The answer is b.** Allotropes are different forms of the same element. Diamonds and graphite are made from carbon. Other examples of allotropes are ozone and oxygen gas, which are allotropes of oxygen.

45.   **The answer is B.** Balancing equations is quite tricky and requires lots of practice to master. On examination of the first substance, we see that methane gas has one carbon atom. There is also one carbon atom on the right side of the equation. There is no need to balance this. There are four hydrogen atoms on the left side. To balance this, we change the coefficients so that there are four hydrogen atoms on the right. This is done by placing a 2 in front of water:

$$\_CH_4 + \_O_2 \rightarrow \_CO_2 + 2H_2O$$

Inspection of the oxygen atoms shows just two atoms of oxygen on the left but a total of four oxygen atoms on the right (two from the water and two from the carbon dioxide). We change the coefficient of the oxygen gas to a 2 so that there are four oxygen atoms on the left. Now the equation is balanced:

$$1CH_4 + 2O_2 \rightarrow CO_2 + 2H_2O$$

46.   **The answer is a.** The nephron's job is to filter the blood that enters the kidney. The ureter, also part of the excretory system, allows urine to exit the body.

47.   **The answer is a.** The cones in the eye are responsible for distinguishing between colors. People who are color-blind have defects in the cones and usually cannot see shades of green and red.

48.   **The answer is a.** Vertebrates have a spinal column, or backbone. A starfish is an invertebrate because it lacks this structure.

49.   **The answer is c.** Capillaries are one cell thick so that gas exchange can take place easily.

50.   **The answer is a.** The atria of the heart receive blood from other parts of the body. The left atrium receives oxygenated blood from the pulmonary veins, whereas the right atrium receives deoxygenated blood from the body.

51.   **The answer is c.** A synapse is the space between neurons. Neurotransmitters travel across this area so that one neuron can communicate with another.

52.   **The answer is b.** The number 1,000,000, or one million, has six zeros, making it 10^6.

53.   **The answer is a.** The number 6,180 meters can be rewritten as 6.180×10^3.

54. **The answer is d**. The prefix *milli-* means one-thousandth and *centi-* means one-hundredth. The prefixes differ by one power of 10. Because the prefix *milli-* is a smaller unit than *centi-*, 10 millimeters are in one centimeter.

55. **The answer is c**. The atomic number of Ar is 18. Subtracting 18 protons from its mass number of 40 gives 22; Ar-40 has 22 neutrons in its nucleus.

56. **The answer is b**. Aluminum as an atom has 13 electrons. The aluminum ion with a +3 charge indicates that the atom lost three electrons and now has 10 electrons.

57. **The answer is c**. Eighteen electrons can be held in principal energy level number three.

58. **The answer is c**. Chlorophyll absorbs red and blue light best; 665 nm corresponds to red light, whereas 430 nm corresponds to blue light.

59. **The answer is a**. The xylem of the plant carries materials from the roots, upward throughout the plant.

60. **The answer is d**. When placed in distilled water, a cell has a higher concentration of solutes inside and a very low concentration of solutes outside. In an effort to dilute the concentration of solutes inside the cell, water flows into the cell, causing it to swell and possibly burst.

Practice Test 5
Verbal Ability Word Knowledge

1. **The answer is b**. To implicate is to show or imply that someone is involved.

2. **The answer is d**. Someone who was fastidious, or demanding, would be a difficult boss.

3. **The answer is a**. In other words, the rumors started as simple gossip but became more sinister or damaging over time.

4. **The answer is b**. In Latin, *dict* means "to speak," as in *dictate* or *dictionary*.

5. **The answer is c**. A crevasse refers to a large crack or separation, often in an ice field such as a glacier.

6. **The answer is a**. The opposite of the big city would be the provinces.

7. **The answer is d**. A gauntlet is a glove, which a knight of old threw down to challenge an opponent.

8. **The answer is b**. The prefix *in-* means "opposite," and *–vert* means "to turn."

9. **The answer is a**. Since her previous employees were obnoxious, she wants someone more pleasant, or amiable.

10. **The answer is c**. Archaically, this refers to pulling a hood or blindfold over someone's eyes. Now it refers to any kind of trickery.

11. **The answer is a**. *Apprehensive* can mean "quick to apprehend," but its more common meaning has to do with anxiety over the future.

12. **The answer is c**. A sanction can be a formal restriction or an authorization.

13. **The answer is a**. Someone who is morose is sad and withdrawn.

14. **The answer is a**. Think of *incredible*, which means "unbelievable." Someone who is credulous believes everything.

15. **The answer is a**. If someone is orderly, they put things in order.

16. **The answer is b**. The roots are *com*, meaning "with" and *laborare*, meaning "to work."

Reading Comprehension

Passage 1

17. **The answer is d**. Hunting and habitat destruction are the only reasons mentioned for the depopulation of elk prior to the twentieth century.

18. **The answer is d**. According to the passage, in 1913, 50 elk were moved from Yellowstone to Pennsylvania. Two years later, 95 more were moved. The total shipped in those years comes to 145.

19. **The answer is d**. "At present," says the passage, "new herds are established in Arkansas, Kentucky, Michigan, and Wisconsin in addition to Pennsylvania."

20. **The answer is b**. As the passage states clearly, "All of the eastern subspecies are now extinct." The reintroduced subspecies is the western subspecies, the one found in Yellowstone. It is a different subspecies from the original Pennsylvania elk.

21. **The answer is c**. Because reintroduction now includes careful monitoring of species and more concern about the animals' welfare, you can infer that the author believes it has improved.

22. **The answer is d**. The work going on in Jackson County shows an example of monitoring that is taking place today.

Passage 2

23. **The answer is b.** The connection between coffee and miscarriage is fully discussed while the others are either not mentioned or minor issues.

24. **The answer is c.** Where the caffeine came from and when it was ingested are irrelevant, according to the passage.

25. **The answer is a.** The answer is found in paragraph 4.

26. **The answer is b.** The findings of the study run counter to the established guidelines of the American College of Obstetricians and Gynecologists, so if accepted, the findings would invalidate those guidelines.

27. **The answer is d.** Some physicians will regard this study as conclusive and change their recommendations, whereas others will wait for more research.

28. **The answer is d.** Posing health risks for some people is the only conclusion that is supported by the passage.

Passage 3

29. **The answer is c.** Survival times are the core of the article.

30. **The answer is c.** The first sentence clearly states this.

31. **The answer is d.** The numbers of those at risk adds urgency and need to this study.

32. **The answer is a.** The researchers are trying to determine the exact longevity of patients with the disease.

33. **The answer is b.** The author states in the last paragraph that the weak and frail died first.

34. **The answer is c.** The irony is that those patients will die before the study's conclusions can help them.

Passage 4

35. **The answer is c.** This is the one choice that fits the entire passage.

36. **The answer is a.** This is the only choice that directly shows the dangers of hospitals.

37. **The answer is d.** The passage says that Lifewings Partners requires its client hospitals "to change their medical and communication procedures, train their doctors and nurses, and establish checklists and measurements designed to track outcomes."

38. **The answer is b.** In the final paragraph of the passage, Lifewings Partners' CEO is quoted as follows: "Just because a hospital has a great reputation for cutting-edge medicine doesn't necessarily mean the hospital is the safest place to go for routine procedures." From this, you can conclude that medical mistakes can happen at even the finest hospitals.

39. **The answer is b.** Context clues are very important here to understand the correct meaning. In this passage, the word *watchdog* is used to mean an organization that watches health care procedures and guards against medical errors.

40. **The answer is c.** Lifewing Partners "works to educate patients on safety before they even enter the hospital."

Passage 5

41. **The answer is b.** The new study indicates that previous anecdotal evidence was correct: Amphibians really *are* barometers of environmental health.

42. **The answer is d.** The answer may be inferred from the opening paragraph, which thanks the scientists involved for offering "proof of this hypothesis" through their "concerted, Internet-based efforts."

43. **The answer is c.** Paragraph 4 includes the information "the highest percentages of threatened species are in the Caribbean," followed by three examples: "In Haiti for example, nine out of ten species of amphibians are threatened. In Jamaica, it is eight out of ten, and in Puerto Rico, seven out of ten."

44. **The answer is b.** The point of the paragraph is to indicate what qualities amphibians have that put them at risk.

45. **The answer is a.** The passage has to do with amphibians and how susceptible they are to environmental degradation. Statistics on numbers of species in Haiti, where amphibians are apparently under siege, might provide strong evidence for the author's contentions.

46. **The answer is c.** The author is warning that amphibians are only the first of all animals to be affected by climate change.

Word Knowledge

47. **The answer is a.** A harangue is a long, scolding speech.

48. **The answer is c.** An achievement is an accomplishment.

49. **The answer is a.** A catalyst is any substance or stimulus that causes things to happen.

50. **The answer is a.** Someone who is affable makes others feel good.

51. **The answer is d.** None of the other choices have to do with a form of payment.

52. **The answer is a.** If the investor is unbelievable, he is likely to be an imposter.

53. **The answer is d.** In Latin the root *viv* means "life"; someone who is vivacious is lively or animated.

54. **The answer is b.** To be pristine is to be unspoiled.

55. **The answer is a.** An incursion is a brief raid, an undesired invasion.

56. **The answer is c.** An untamed hawk is a haggard, but the word is more frequently used to mean having an untamed or wild look.

57. **The answer is a.** Ephemera are things that don't last very long, such as a vapor cloud. To dissipate is to scatter or dissolve.

58. **The answer is b.** Niccolo Machiavelli wrote a book about how to be cunning in politics.

59. **The answer is d.** To exacerbate is to make more intense, as in pain, irritation, or trouble.

60. **The answer is a.** You can see the roots of the word *joke* in the adjective *jocund*.

Mathematics

1. **The answer is b.** Cross-multiply to get:

    $(56)(8) = (4x + 8)(1)$

    $448 = 4x + 8$

    Subtract 8 from both sides to get:

    $440 = 4x$

    Divide both sides by 4 to get: $110 = x$

2. **The answer is a.** The equation is in the form of a quadratic equation $ax^2 + bx + c = 0$, where $a = 1$, $b = -2$, and $c = -1$. To solve this problem, you use the quadratic formula or

    $$\frac{-b \pm \sqrt{b^2 - 4ac}}{2a}.$$

3. **The answer is c.** The sum of $\left(\frac{4}{3}\right)^2 + \left(\frac{2}{4}\right)^2$ can be found by first computing the value of each term.

$$\left(\frac{4}{3}\right)^2 = \left(\frac{4^2}{3^2}\right) = \frac{16}{9}$$

$$\left(\frac{2}{4}\right)^2 = \left(\frac{2^2}{4^2}\right) = \frac{4}{16} = \frac{1}{4}$$

$$\left(\frac{4}{3}\right)^2 + \left(\frac{2}{4}\right)^2 = \frac{16}{9} + \frac{1}{4} = \frac{64}{36} + \frac{9}{36} = \frac{73}{36}.$$

4. **The answer is c.** From the first equation, multiply both sides by y, resulting in $x = 8y$.

Because $x = 64$, you can write

$$64 = 8y$$

or $\quad y = \frac{64}{8} = 8$

Substituting the given information regarding x and y into its sum yields:

$$x + y = 64 + 8 = 72.$$

5. **The answer is d.** The probability of not getting a 2 on the roll of the dice can be found using the equation $q = \frac{f}{n} = n - \frac{s}{n} - s$, where n is the total number of possible outcomes ($n = 6$) and s is the number of outcomes considered a success ($s = 1$). So $q = -n - \frac{s}{n} = 6 - \frac{1}{6} = \frac{5}{6}$.

Another way of looking at this problem would be that the probability of not rolling a 2 is equal to the probability of rolling a 1, 3, 4, 5, and 6, which is five out of a possible six outcomes.

6. **The answer is b.** To determine the probability that a selected card is a 10, you should first note that a card can be selected from a deck in $n = 52$ different ways. Since there are four 10 cards, one 10 for each of the four suits, a 10 can be drawn from the deck in $s = 4$ different ways. Thus, the probability that the selected card is a 10 is: $p = \frac{s}{n} = \frac{4}{52} = \frac{1}{13}$.

7. **The answer is b.** A little translation is a big help on this problem: The question "8 is what percent of 5?" translates to "$8 = \frac{x}{100} \times 5$." To solve, $8 \times 100 = \frac{5x}{100} \times 100$, which comes out to $800 = 5x$, which becomes $\frac{800}{5} = \frac{5x}{5}$ or $160 = x$.

8. **The answer is b.** The product must be less than $300 \times 30 + 300 \times 5$, which is 10,500. Choice a is way too low and choices c and d are way too high.

9. **The correct choice is b**. 18 is divisible by 2, 3, 6, and 9, other than itself and 1; 21 is divisible by 3 and 7; 25 is divisible by 5.

10. **The answer is b**. Converting a percent to a decimal just involves removing the percent sign and moving the decimal point two places to the left. Therefore, 65% becomes 0.65.

11. **The answer is b**. This problem uses a Pythagorean shortcut, but you can also use the Pythagorean theorem if you forget the shortcuts. The sides of the rectangle are 5 and 12, so you can plug those numbers into the theorem and get $5^2 + 12^2 = c^2$. That brings you to $169 = c^2$ or $\sqrt{169} = c^2$, which solves as $13 = c$.

12. **The answer is d**. You are looking for 20%, or $\frac{1}{5}$ of the pie chart, which has a degree measure of 360. $\frac{1}{5} \times 360$ is 72.

13. **The answer is c**. $(94 + 91 + 88 + 95) \div 4 = 92$; therefore, Polly's average on the four tests was 92.

14. **The answer is c**. If a problem has exponents of the same base being multiplied, you *add* the exponents: $7^3 \times 7^5 = 7^8$.

15. **The answer is a**. One way to do this problem is to reduce the answer choices until you find one that equals 15:8, which choice a does. Another way is to set the answer choices up as proportions with 15:8, and bowtie to compare them. The one that comes out with equal numbers on both sides is the equal ratio.

16. **The answer is b**. $(3 + 14 + 10 + -7) \div 4 = 5$; therefore, the average of the list of numbers is 5.

17. **The answer is d**. Because the question is asking for a prime number, you can immediately eliminate the even answer choices, a and c. The number 27 is not prime because it is divisible by 3, and 29 is prime.

18. **The answer is d**. The answer choices with absolute value signs must be positive, so to find the largest value, pick the largest positive number, which is 7.2.

19. **The answer is b**. You would need to look for the smallest angle of incline in the line.

20. **The answer is b**. February and April both show an increase of more than 10°; they each increase by about 12 or 13.

21. **The answer is b**. 9 from 12 is 3, but of the two answers that start with 3, only one is close.

22. **The answer is c**. You are asked to determine the probability of randomly selecting one face card (king, queen, or jack) of a spade suit from two standard decks of cards. Because there are two decks of cards, a single card can be selected from

two decks in $n = 104$ different ways. Since there are three face cards of a spade suit in one deck of cards, such a card can be drawn from the two decks in $s = 6$ different ways. Thus, the probability that the selected card is a face card of a spade suit is: $p = p = \dfrac{s}{n} = \dfrac{6}{104}$.

23. **The answer is b.** The number 46 is not prime. However, 47 is prime, making it the smallest prime number in the answer choices.

24. **The answer is b.** The total amount of degrees $(40° + 30°)$ can be written as a fraction of the total number of degrees in a circle $(360°)$. $\dfrac{60}{360} = \dfrac{1}{6}$. Convert the fraction to a decimal: $\dfrac{1}{6} = 0.1666$. Rounding this to the nearest whole percent is 17%.

25. **The answer is c.** The other choices are irrational numbers that cannot be expressed as fractions. They are real numbers but they are nonterminating, non-repeating numbers. The set of rational numbers includes all integers and common fractions like those shown on the number line.

26. **The answer is b.** The prime factors of 56 are 2, 2, 2, and 7. One pair of twos can come outside the radical, and the other 2 and the 7 must stay in.

27. **The answer is b.** An interpretation of the data shows that substantially fewer admissions came from South and there has to be a reason for this. Emergency rooms are chosen by how close by they are when a person is sick. The other interpretations of data are incorrect, and this is provable by the number of admissions from each region.

28. **The answer is c.** The formula for the perimeter of a rectangle is $P = 2l + 2w$. In this case: $2 \times 5 + 2 \times 3 = 16$. Measurements of area would show m² because of multiplication, not addition.

29. **The answer is d.** The point is both negative and positive. Negative on the x-axis and positive on the y-axis.

30. **The answer is d.** You can see that to find the missing quantity, you would have to subtract $2\dfrac{4}{5}$ from the whole. $6 - 2\dfrac{4}{5} = \dfrac{6}{1} - \dfrac{14}{5}$. Multiplying across gives you 30 – 14 for the numerator and 5 for the denominator, so that is a complete fraction of $\dfrac{16}{5}$ or $3\dfrac{1}{5}$, if the question has mixed numbers.

31. **The correct choice is d.**
    $45 = (125\%)x$
    $45 = (1.25)x$
    $36 = x$

32. **The correct choice is c.** This question is asking for the area of a rectangle, so you just need to multiply the sides; $18 \times 12 = 216$.

33. **The answer is c.** In January, the column for 8–15 is in the middle, either 22 or 23. In February, it is also in the middle, either 17 or 18. So you know the number of 8- to 15-year-old patients is between 39 and 41.

34. **The answer is a.** This time you are focusing on just the January numbers, in black. It looks like the 1–7 column is almost all the way to the 15 line, so call it 14. The patients 16–23 column is almost all the way to the 10 line, so call it 9, giving you a difference of about 5, which is choice a; no other answer comes close.

35. **The answer is a.** To solve the inequality $2x - 3 > 3 - 4x$, you need to collect like terms of x on one side of the inequality and all other values to the other side. First add 3 to both sides of the inequality:

    $2x - 3 + 3 > 3 - 4x + 3$
    $2x > 6 - 4x$

    Then add $4x$ to both sides of the inequality:

    $2x + 4x > 6 - 4x + 4x$
    $6x > 6$

    Dividing both sides by 6 yields $x > 1$.

36. **The answer is b.** Multiply both sides by $3x + 42$ so $24 = \frac{2}{9} \times 3x + 42$. Multiply both sides by $\frac{9}{2}$ (the reciprocal of $\frac{2}{9}$). So $\frac{9}{2} \times 24 = 3x + 42$ and $108 = 3x + 42$.

    $108 - 42 = 3x$
    $66 = 3x$
    $22 = x$

37. **The answer is d.** From the first equation, multiply both sides by y, resulting in $x = 5y$. Because $x = 25$, you can write

    $25 = 5y$

    or $\quad y = \frac{25}{5} = 5.$

    Substituting the given information regarding x and y into its sum yields:

    $x + y = 25 + 5 = 30.$

38. **The answer is a.** To determine the quotient of $(6x^3y^4z^2)$ divided by $(2xy^3z^5)$, the two monomials as a division problem with one expression on top of another:

    $$\frac{(6x^3y^4z^2)}{(2xy^3z^5)} = \left(\frac{6}{2}\right)\left(\frac{x^3}{x}\right)\left(\frac{y^4}{y^3}\right)\left(\frac{z^2}{z^5}\right) = 3 \times x^2 \times y \times z^{-3} = \frac{3x^2y}{z^3}.$$

39. **The answer is c.** Given the equation $\dfrac{x^2-4x-21}{x+3}=1$, you must first try to simplify the numerator by expressing the polynomial in terms of its factors or $\dfrac{x^2-4x+21}{x+3}=\dfrac{(x-7)(x+3)}{x+3}=1$. The term $(x+3)$ can be eliminated from the numerator and denominator because any term divided by itself is 1. Thus, the equation above can be simplified as: $(x-7)=1$ or $x=8$.

40. **The answer is c.** When asked to solve an absolute value equation, it is helpful to write the equation in its two forms:

    (1) $2x-4=20$

    (2) $2x-4=-20$

    Solving for x in equation (1) yields $x=12$ and in equation (2) yields $x=-8$.

Science

1. **The answer is b.** Cytokinesis literally means "cytoplasm movement." This occurs during telophase and is the final phase of cell replication.

2. **The answer is a.** Carnivores are meat eaters, whereas herbivores are plant eaters. Consumers are organisms that eat others, and decomposers help decay materials so that they can be recycled in the environment.

3. **The answer is b.** During metaphase, the chromosomes line up near the equator of the cell in preparation for the separation of the chromosomes and the pinching of the cytoplasm.

4. **The answer is a.** The term *lysis* means "to split." The enzymes in lysosomes break down substrates into desired products.

5. **The answer is a.** The lock-and-key model describes how the substrate must fit into the active site of an enzyme for the reaction to take place.

6. **The answer is d.** Organisms that contain chlorophyll are most likely green.

7. **The answer is a.** Water has a density of 1 g/mL. To float, the object must have a density that is less than that of water. The object labeled W floats and objects X, Y, and Z sink.

8. **The answer is b.** For the substance to decay from 40 grams to 10 grams it must undergo two half-lives (40 → 20 → 10). If it takes 16 days for two half-lives to occur, it takes just 8 days for one half-life to occur.

9. **The answer is d.** To become a female, each parent must give an X chromosome so that there are two X chromosomes present. The mother of the human fetus always gives an X chromosome, whereas the father can provide either an X or Y. Because the variation lies with the father, the father's sperm determines the sex of the fetus.

10. **The answer is a.** The sun provides plants with the energy to grow. It is the producers who serve as the basis for the food that other organisms consume.

11. **The answer is c.** Both lipids and carbohydrates contain carbon, oxygen, and hydrogen. Although both proteins and nucleic acids contain nitrogen, only the nucleic acid has a phosphate group.

12. **The answer is a.** Leukocytes are white blood cells that identify pathogens and attack them. Stem cells are immature cells that can replace lost cells. The spleen is an organ that controls the amount of blood in the body and eliminates old blood cells. Bone marrow produces white blood cells and stem cells.

13. **The answer is c.** Cilia are small hairs inside the nasal passage that help clear dirt and other particles so they don't go into the lungs. The epiglottis is not in the nose but in the throat and is a flap of tissue that covers the vocal cords to protect them from food when you are eating. The external meatus is the fleshy object in the center of the face shaped like a triangle that is commonly referred to as the nose. The tonsils are part of the lymphatic system and protect the body after infection.

14. **The answer is b.** Although a snake is very flexible, it has a backbone, which makes it a vertebrate. All the others lack a true backbone.

15. **The answer is d.** A sound's pitch is determined by how quickly the source of the sound vibrates or its frequency. The Doppler effect describes changes in frequency caused by the movement of a sound source. Decibels measure the intensity of a sound wave, not its loudness. Ultrasonic describes sound waves that are beyond human perception.

16. **The answer is c.** The right atrium receives oxygen-poor blood from the body and pumps it into the right ventricle, and from there it goes to the lungs. The left atrium receives oxygen-rich blood from the lungs and pumps it into left ventricle, which sends it out to the body.

17. **The answer is a.** When an acid and a base react, water is produced and salt remains. The metal in a salt comes from the base and the nonmetal part comes from the acid. A gel is a colloid in which long particles trap a liquid inside.

18. **The answer is b.** Atoms with more protons in the nucleus have a greater nuclear charge than atoms with fewer protons.

19. **The answer is a**. The initial sample starts with 100 grams. Because the half-life is five days, every five days only half of the sample will remain. After the first five days only 50 grams will remain. Because the problem calls for the mass after 10 days, in another five days only 25 grams of the original sample will remain. This process can be outlined as follows:

    100 grams – 5 days → 50 grams – 5 more days (10 days total) → 25 grams

20. **The answer is d**. The reaction $^{232}_{90}\text{Th} \rightarrow \,^{228}_{88}\text{Ra} + \text{X}$ shows that a particle was produced as a result of nuclear decay. This transmutation shows an original mass number of 232 before the reaction and 228 after the reaction. This is a loss of 4 AMU. The number of protons before the decay was 90 and it became 88 after the decay, resulting in a net loss of two protons.

21. **The answer is b**. Neon has 10 electrons. This is a configuration of 2–8.

22. **The answer is b**. The modern periodic table is arranged by atomic number.

23. **The answer is a**. The nonmetals are located in the upper right of the periodic table.

24. **The answer is d**. Elements in the same group/family are chemically similar. Mg and Ca are in the same group on the periodic table.

25. **The answer is b**. Carbon has 6 protons.

26. **The answer is c**. Oxygen has 8 protons.

27. **The answer is c**. Carbon has 8 neutrons. Subtracting the number of protons from the mass number gives the number of neutrons: 8 for carbon-14.

28. **The answer is d**. Fluorine has the highest electronegativity. Because iodine (I) is the element farthest from fluorine (F), it has the lowest electronegativity of the choices.

29. **The answer is a**. Fluorine and neon are nonmetals and are expected to have smaller atomic radii because they are located next to each other on the periodic table. Because strontium is located on the lower left of the periodic table, it has a larger atomic radius than cobalt.

30. **The answer is b**. Aluminum is a metal. Further proof lies in the aluminum pan in your kitchen, which is shiny and conducts heat.

31. **The answer is a**. The compound CO is formed from two nonmetals and is a covalent compound.

32. **The answer is d**. Potassium (K) is a metal, and iodine (I) is a nonmetal. This means that an ionic compound forms. To do this, the metal K loses an electron to the nonmetal I.

33. **The answer is c.** All of the compounds listed are covalently bonded because they contain all nonmetals. The equal sharing occurs when the electronegativity of the elements is the same.

34. **The answer is b.** Proteins, lipids, nucleic acids, and carbohydrates are the four major organic compounds that are important to living things. Synthetic polymers, although they can be placed into living things, are not formed by the body naturally.

35. **The answer is a.** Glucose is a simple sugar and is what carbohydrates and starches need to be turned into so that they can be used by cells.

36. **The answer is d.** The wavelike movement of muscles in the digestive system is called peristalsis. This pushes food through the digestive tract.

37. **The answer is c.** Atherosclerosis is the hardening of the arteries. As cholesterol builds up, the opening in the artery closes, leading to a heart attack.

38. **The answer is b.** The esophagus connects the mouth to the stomach. The epiglottis covers the glottis so that food does not enter the windpipe or lungs. The anus allows the release of fecal matter from the body.

39. **The answer is a.** Cellular respiration includes the other three processes; glucose is broken down into other substances in a number of different processes. The processes have one goal, to produce the ATP needed by our cells.

40. **The answer is d.** The chlorophyll in plants absorbs red and blue light best.

41. **The answer is c.** The scientific name of an organism includes its genus and species.

42. **The answer is c.** Insects are classified as herbivores because they eat plants. This is not to be confused with producers, which are the green plants.

43. **The answer is b.** For the plant to be short, it must have alleles that are tt. For the plant to be tall, it must have alleles Tt or TT. Crossing Tt with tt gives the following: Tt, Tt, tt, and tt. This cross demonstrates that 50% of the plants are short.

44. **The answer is c.** Photosynthesis creates glucose and oxygen gas from carbon dioxide, water, and light energy. Respiration takes oxygen gas and glucose to make energy, carbon dioxide, and water.

45. **The answer is b.** Flowers have the organs that are responsible for sexual reproduction. The male reproductive organs are called stamens, and the female reproductive organs are called pistils.

46. **The answer is a.** The melting of ice requires the ice to absorb heat, an endothermic process.

47. **The answer is c.** The reaction synthesizes water from hydrogen and oxygen. The reaction also indicates the release of heat energy—an exothermic reaction.

48. **The answer is d**. Fluorine has been labeled as a gas, which is the phase that is most easily compressed.

49. **The answer is a**. The compound $I_2(s)$ indicates solid iodine, which has a definite shape and volume.

50. **The answer is a**. Portion BC of the graph shows a phase change and no temperature change. Because it is occurring at the melting point of the substance, this is where the solid and liquid phase will exist together.

51. **The answer is c**. Graham's law takes into account masses of gases and their speed. The other three choices all take into account the volume, pressure, and temperature of a sample of gas.

52. **The answer is b**. Monosaccharides, such as glucose, can join to form long molecules called starches. Amino acids would form proteins, and nucleic acids would form DNA and RNA.

53. **The answer is d**. Catalysts are not consumed or altered during a chemical reaction. Catalysts lower the activation energy of a reaction and then proceed to carry out this process again and again, without being destroyed.

54. **The answer is d**. The rectum stores fecal matter before it is eliminated from the body. The mouth, small intestine, and stomach all have gastric juices containing enzymes to digest foods.

55. **The answer is b**. The atomic mass of nitrogen is 14.0 and the atomic mass of a hydrogen atom is 1.0. Because there are three hydrogen atoms, it is necessary to add 14.0 and 3.0, which gives 17.0.

56. **The answer is a**. CaO has a gram formula mass of 56 because the atomic mass of Ca is 40 and the gram atomic mass of oxygen is 16.

57. **The answer is c**. A spike in FSH and LH occur during ovulation as a follicle in the ovary ruptures and releases an egg into the fallopian tube.

58. **The answer is c**. The bladder (3) stores urine produced in the kidney (1) and is transported from the kidney to the bladder by the ureter (2). From the bladder, the urethra passes urine to the outside.

59. **The correct answer is b**. The general trend in ionization energy for atoms across a period is that the ionization energy increases from left to right. The trend in a column is that the ionization energy increases from the bottom to the top of a column. The trend across a period means that O < F. The trend in the column means that S < O. Putting these two results together gives S < O < F. For cations, the ionization energy is always greater than that of the atom from which the cation is derived, so F < F^+, giving a final order of S < O < F < F^+.

60. **The answer is a.** Chlorine is element number 17, so its atom must have 17 electrons. This rules out choices c and d, which have 18 electrons. Choice b is the ground state electron configuration of Cl. Choice a has one of the 3p electrons promoted to the higher 3d level. This is the correct answer.

Practice Test 6

Verbal Ability Word Knowledge and Reading Comprehension

1. **The answer is a.** Adjacent and alongside are synonyms.

2. **The answer is c.** *Bene* in Latin means "good" or, in this case, "successful."

3. **The answer is b.** The opposite of expensive is a loss of value, or depreciation.

4. **The answer is b.** After six days, anyone would be starving or ravenous.

5. **The answer is c.** *Sub* means "below" in Latin, so subservient would mean to lower yourself or be submissive and docile.

6. **The answer is a.** Showing discretion means you know when to stay quiet about something embarrassing.

7. **The answer is b.** Vitriol is an ancient name for sulfuric acid, which is caustic and bitter or acerbic.

8. **The answer is c.** Something inscrutable cannot be read, such as a person's facial expression.

9. **The answer is d.** Stating your opinion with emphasis shows your boss you stand behind your beliefs and you are not obsequious.

10. **The answer is b.** If you are pretending to be something you are not, you are being pretentious.

11. **The answer is a.** Something immaculate is spotless, so guests who have impeccable manners are beyond reproach.

12. **The answer is b.** In Latin, *pugnare* means "to fight," so this dog is a fighter.

13. **The answer is d.** *Metropolitan* means "Greek," so *cosmopolitan* means "citizen of the world," or well-traveled. She can see many or diverse viewpoints from traveling.

14. **The answer is c.** From the Greek, *auto* means "one's self" or "control," so a robot has control of itself.

15. **The answer is a.** *Frugal* comes from "fruit," as in having a good harvest by saving money and being practical.

16. **The answer is d.** The Latin root of *tumult* is "disorder" or "chaos."

Reading Comprehension

Passage 1

17. **The answer is c.** The angel's glow phenomenon was unexplained for decades.

18. **The answer is a.** The inference is that a divine explanation was necessary.

19. **The answer is d.** He had to narrow his search to blue light, as this was the only big clue.

20. **The answer is b.** This is stated in paragraph 3.

21. **The answer is a.** The other choices are unlikely outcomes.

22. **The answer is d.** This conclusion is explained by the fact that cold kills the bacteria.

Passage 2

23. **The answer is a.** The author discusses good and bad ancient medical practices.

24. **The answer is b.** The other statements are plainly false, and the author is being evenhanded.

25. **The answer is c.** The idea of testing proves medicine that really works.

26. **The answer is d.** This term is defined in paragraph 1.

27. **The answer is d.** You have to extrapolate the idea of how ancient doctors should experiment carefully to cure people.

28. **The answer is d.** Mercury took the man's life because he wanted to receive eternal life from the poisonous mineral.

Passage 3

29. **The answer is c.** The allure of glitter covers all the ways it is discussed.

30. **The answer is a.** This is stated in paragraph 3.

31. **The answer is c.** The law was designed to keep the oceans clean.

32. **The answer is d.** This conclusion comes from the fact stated that companies won't say if their product has glitter because they fear backlash.

33. **The answer is b.** This is stated in paragraph 3.

34. **The answer is b.** The other inferences are unsupported by the selection.

Passage 4

35. **The answer is c.** It is about the general problem of polio and controlling it.

36. **The answer is a.** The vaccine kept people from being infected, solving all problems.

37. **The answer is d.** The emphasis on eradicating all polio shows its virility.

38. **The answer is c.** The author stresses attacking polio worldwide.

39. **The answer is b.** This choice is the most supported and the focus of the selection.

40. **The answer is b.** The idea that it got suddenly worse is crucial to understanding why a vaccine was desperately needed.

Passage 5

41. **The answer is d.** While the others are all mentioned, the focus is on ballooning.

42. **The answer is a.** Electrical flight is the cause; the other choices are lesser facts.

43. **The answer is b.** Without circulation, they couldn't fly, so they have to use other means.

44. **The answer is c.** In paragraph 5, trichobothria is defined.

45. **The answer is a.** Unknown skills of other organisms are discussed, making this inference correct.

46. **The answer is c.** The experiment described proved what scientists had seen but were only guessing about.

Word Knowledge

47. **The answer is d.** *Im-* or *in-* means "into," so something absorbed or immersed is placed inside or hidden from the outside, such as a surgeon concentrating on his work.

48. **The answer is b.** A sacred place offers sanctuary or a safe place.

49. **The answer is a.** The prefixes *e-* or *ex-* are Latin meaning "out," so to eradicate or exterminate is to wipe out or kill.

50. **The answer is c.** Being turned away from a straight path describes direction and a child who doesn't obey society's norms.

51. **The answer is d.** A failed water sanitation system would be a disaster.

52. **The answer is d.** Again, Latin *ex-* means "out" or "off," so to forgive someone is to let them off.

53. **The answer is c.** A diatribe was originally a discussion or lecture, but today it means lengthy criticism.

54. **The answer is a.** The prefix *co-* or *com-* means "stick," as in adhere or people sticking together.

55. **The answer is a.** In Greek, a *myriad* was 10,000 or any large number.

56. **The answer is d.** Being poorly dressed makes you a *sloven*, or a messy person.

57. **The answer is c.** High energy usually means noise and activity.

58. **The answer is b.** *Serene* indicates a clear thought and peacefulness.

59. **The answer is a.** *Ex-* again means "out" and is joined with *thought* to mean well thought out or excellent.

60. **The answer is d.** The prefix *mal-* indicates something bad.

Mathematics

1. **The answer is b.** To determine the percent increase, convert the percentage shown to a decimal by dividing by 100. Then multiply the existing amount by that decimal.

$$\frac{18\%}{100} = 0.18$$
$$3900 \times 0.18 = 702$$

Now add this amount to the existing daily cost.

$702 + 3900 = \$4,602$ This will be the new average cost in 10 years.

2. **The answer is d.** Dividing a negative integer by another negative integer will result in a positive quotient.

$-36 \div -6 =$ Perform the division without signs.

$36 \div 6 = 6$ Then determine if the quotient should be positive or negative.

$+6$ Both dividend and divisor were negative so the quotient will be positive.

3. **The answer is b.** You have to convert minutes to seconds in order to solve this problem. Create a proportion using the given information and substitute x for the unknown pulse rate. Make sure that the number of beats is the numerator and that the time frames are the denominator on both sides of the equal sign.

$$\frac{90 \text{ beats}}{60 \text{ seconds}} = \frac{x \text{ beats}}{20 \text{ seconds}}$$ Cross-multiply.

$60x = 1,800$ Divide both sides by 60 for x.

$x = 30$

4. **The answer is a.** You have to factor 63 because it does not have a whole-number square root.

$\sqrt{63} = \sqrt{9 \cdot 7}$ Rewrite each factor with its own square root symbol.

$\sqrt{9} \cdot \sqrt{7} = \sqrt{63}$ Factor 9. 7 is a prime number.

$\sqrt{3} \cdot \sqrt{7} =$ Simplify.

$3\sqrt{7} = \sqrt{63}$

5. **The answer is a.** Look for common factors that appear in both the numerator and denominator. You need to isolate like elements. Note that both have squares of x and y, as well as multiplying each other.

$$\frac{x^2 + xy}{y^2 + xy} = \frac{x(x - y)}{y(y - x)}$$

Now make both expressions within the parentheses equal by factoring out −1 in the denominator.

$$\frac{x(x - y)}{y(y - x)} = \frac{x(x - y)}{y(-1)(-y + x)} = \frac{x(x - y)}{-y(x - y)}$$

Next, in both the numerator and the denominator, divide out the $(x - y)$.

$$\frac{x(x - y)}{-y(x - y)} = -\frac{x}{y}$$ which becomes $-\frac{x}{y}$.

6. **The answer is b.** You will need to align units across from unit and milliliters across from milliliters using a proportion in order to solve this problem.

$$\frac{1,200,000 \text{ units}}{\text{ml}} = \frac{80,000 \text{ units}}{x}$$ Multiply across the fraction, units and ml.

$$1,200,000x = 80,000$$ Divide both sides by 1,200,000 to find x.

$$x = \frac{80,000}{1,200,000} = \frac{8}{12} = \frac{2}{3} \text{ ml.}$$

7. **The answer is a.** Here you know the percent and the percentage and need to find the base with an equation that states their relationship.

$$96 = 80\% \cdot x$$ Convert the percentage by dividing by 100, then multiplying.
$$96 = 0.80 \, x$$

$$\frac{96}{0.80} = \frac{0.80x}{0.80}$$
$$120 = x$$

8. **The answer is d.** A period of half a day is 12 hours. If the temperature rose 0.25 every hour, you would multiply 12×0.25. This would be a total increase of 3.0°F. Her original temperature was 101.7. Be sure to line up the decimal place values appropriately.

101.7
+ 3.0
104.7

9. **The answer is a.** First, you have to deal with the terms inside the parentheses. Multiply these by the −4 outside the parentheses. Note that the integer −4 is right beside the parentheses, thus indicating multiplication of both terms.

$$8 - 4(a - 5b) = 8 + -4a + 20b = 8 - 4a + 20b$$

10. **The answer is d.** You have to convert the fractions within the parentheses in order to complete the addition first. Find a common denominator, which in this case is 8, so $\frac{1}{2}$ becomes $\frac{4}{8}$ and is added to $\frac{1}{8}$ to make $\frac{5}{8}$. Multiply this by $\frac{2}{3}$ to make $\frac{10}{24}$. Reduce this fraction to $\frac{5}{12}$.

$$\frac{2}{3}\left(\frac{1}{2} + \frac{1}{8}\right) =$$

$$\frac{2}{3}\left(\frac{4}{8} + \frac{1}{8}\right) =$$

$$\frac{2}{3} \cdot \frac{5}{8} = \frac{10}{24}$$

$$\frac{10}{24} = \frac{5}{12}$$

11. **The answer is d.** There are 1,000 milliliters in 1 liter, so you would need to multiply 2.74 by 1,000. That would move the decimal point three places to the right.

$2.74 \times 1,000 = 2,740$ milliliters

12. **The answer is d.** In order to solve this problem, you need to apply the formula for determining the volume of a cube: $V = LWH$. In this case, the formula would be stated:

$V = 12 \times 18 \times 10$
$V = 2,160$ cubic m

13. **The answer is c.** In order to solve the problem, simplify all radical expressions.

$\sqrt{72} + \sqrt{18} =$

$\sqrt{4 \cdot 18} + \sqrt{9 \cdot 2} =$ Continue to simplify and factor any integers possible.

$2\sqrt{18} + 3\sqrt{2} =$ Continue simplifying.

$2\sqrt{2 \cdot 9} + 3\sqrt{2} =$

$2(3)\sqrt{2} + 3\sqrt{2} =$ Multiply.

$6\sqrt{2} + 3\sqrt{2} =$ Add like elements.

$9\sqrt{2}$

14. **The answer is d.** A liter is equal to 1,000 milliliters. To calculate what part of a liter that is, you divide 400 milliliters.

$400 \div 1,000 = 0.4$ or $4/10 = 2/5$ of a liter.

15. **The answer is c.** Here you have to convert 12.5 percent to a decimal by dividing by 1,000 based on three placeholders.

$$\frac{12.5}{1,000} = 0.125 = \frac{125}{1,000}$$ Then reduce the fraction to lowest form.

$$\frac{125}{1,000} \div \frac{125}{125} = \frac{1}{8}$$

16. **The answer is a.** In order to solve this problem, the amount of drug per dose has to be calculated.

3×625 mg $= 1,875$ mg   You would then set up a proportion.

$$\frac{1 \text{ mg}}{0.001 \text{ gm}} = \frac{1,875}{x}$$ Cross-multiply to solve for x.

$x = 1.875$ gm   1.875 gm is an overdose, 0.375 gm more than the 1.5-gm limit.

17. **The answer is c.** The formula for determining the area of a triangle is

$$A = \frac{1}{2} \text{ bh}$$

Using the information given, you would create a formula that looks like this:

$A = \frac{1}{2}(3)(6)$ Multiply.

$A = \frac{1}{2}(18)$ Simplify.

$A = 9$ This is the area in meters.

18. **The answer is c.** To solve for b, substitute 5 for a.

$7a = 4b + 11$ becomes $7(5) = 4b + 11$.   Simplify.
$35 = 4b + 11$ Subtract 11 from both sides to isolate b.
$35 - 11 = 4b$ becomes $24 = 4b$.   Divide both sides by 4 to isolate b.
$\frac{24}{4} = \frac{4b}{4}$ becomes $6 = b$.

19. **The answer is c.** Creating a proportion fraction is the easiest way to solve this problem. But first you must divide 1 gram by 1,000 milligrams to convert measurements to like amounts for cross-multiplication.

$$\frac{1 \text{ gm}}{1,000 \text{ mg}} = \frac{1}{0.001 \text{ mg}}$$ Use this form for the proportion.

$$\frac{1}{0.001 \text{ mg}} = \frac{345}{x}$$ Cross-multiply to isolate and define x.

$x = 0.345$ mg

20. **The answer is d.** Create an equation that states the base and the percentage you know.

$x\% \times 265 = 175$ You need to solve for x, the unknown percentage.
$265x = 175$ Multiply x and the base.
$x = \frac{175}{265}$ Divide both sides by 265 to isolate x.

$x = 0.66$ Convert the answer to a percentage by multiplying by 100.

66%

21. **The answer is d.** The decimal points must be lined up properly to keep integers in proper place value. You need to add zeros as placeholders if both decimals are not carried out to the same number of place values.

$$593.100$$
$$\underline{-36.821}$$
$$556.279$$

22. **The answer is a.** You need to convert the total amount of blood donated that day into pints in order to solve the problem. Each quart contains 2 pints of blood. Therefore, multiply 7¼ quarts of blood collected by 2.

$$7\frac{1}{4} \times 2 =$$

$$\frac{29}{4} \cdot \frac{2}{1} =$$

$$\frac{58}{4} = 14\frac{2}{4} \text{ (pints collected)}$$

Now use the pints collected fraction in its unreduced form ($14\frac{2}{4}$) to have common denominators with the amount of blood used after the accident ($3\frac{1}{4}$). Subtract whole numbers as well as numerators.

$$14\frac{2}{4}$$

$$-3\frac{1}{4}$$

$$11\frac{1}{4} \text{ pints}$$

This is the number of pints of blood remaining from the drive.

23. **The answer is c.** Carmen's credits are represented by x. Therefore, Latoya's credits can be represented algebraically as $x + 7$, because she has 7 more credits than Latoya. So, together both women's credits can be expressed as $x + x + 7$. The problem states that they have 82 credits together, so the x's can be combined and written as the equation $2x + 7 = 82$.

24. **The answer is c.** The number 79 is only divisible by 1 or itself. 74 is an even number, 77 can be divided by 7, and 81 is a factor of 9×9.

25. **The answer is d.** Triangles that are similar have proportional sides. They have a constant ratio between corresponding sides. Create a proportion diagram.

$$\frac{\text{6-m side (smaller triangle)}}{\text{12-m side (larger triangle)}} = \frac{\text{8-m side (larger triangle)}}{x}$$ Cross-multiply.

$6x = 96$ Divide both sides by 6.

$x = 16$

26. **The answer is c.** You need only to add the exponents when the bases are the same in order to multiply powers.

$$5z^3 \times 4z^5 = 20z^{3+5} = 20z^8$$

27. **The answer is a.** A ratio is an expression of a relationship between two numbers reduced to their lowest factors to make it easier to understand. The ratio stated in the problem can be written in its most complex form.

330,000 to 3,200,000   This needs to be factored like any fraction not in its simplest form. To do so, state it as a fraction.

$$\frac{330,000}{3,200,000}$$ This fraction can be reduced like any other. Divide both by 330,000.

$$\frac{1}{9.696} \text{ or } \frac{1}{9.7}$$ The denominator can be rounded off to 9.7 or even 10.

The approximate ratio of male to female registered nurses in the United States today is 1:10.

28. **The answer is d.** A whole number percentage like 41 percent means 41 parts out of a hundred parts. So, 0.41 multiplied by 100 equals 41 percent.

29. **The answer is c.** In order to divide fractions with different denominators, invert the second fraction and multiply numerators and denominators.

$$\frac{5}{6} \div \frac{2}{3} = \frac{5}{6} \times \frac{3}{2} = \frac{15}{12}$$

Then reduce by a factor of 3: $\frac{15}{12} = \frac{5}{4} = 1\frac{1}{4}$.

30. **The answer is b.** Compare the denominators after completing each operation. $a = 4$; $b = 32$; $c = 2$; $d = 12$. Note that the numerators are all the same. Therefore, the largest denominator (32) will have the smallest value.

31. **The answer is c.** The easiest way to solve this problem is to create a proportion that states the information as an equation.

$$\frac{\text{8 (right)}}{\text{2 (left)}} = \frac{x}{\text{50 (left)}}$$ Cross-multiply the equation.

$2x = 400$ Divide both sides of the equation by 2.

$x = 200$

32. **The answer is a.** Add the results of contractions from each minute to find a total of 40. Then divide by the total number of results (5) to find the average (8).

33. **The answer is c.** Set up a proportion with the units of mg and ml across from each other.

$$\frac{25 \text{ mg}}{10 \text{ ml}} = \frac{85 \text{ mg}}{x}$$ Cross-multiply.

$25x = 850$ Divide both sides by 25.

$x = 34$ ml

34. **The answer is c.** This is a simple multiplication problem. Convert the percent to a decimal by dividing by 100, and then multiply the base for the percentage.

$29\% \div 100 = 0.29$

$0.29 \times 486 = 140.94$

35. **The answer is d.** Take the total number of beds with patients and multiply it by $\frac{3}{4}$ to determine the number of patients that represent the cutoff point stipulated by hospital policy.

$$24 \cdot \frac{3}{4} = \frac{24}{1} \cdot \frac{3}{4} = \frac{72}{4} = 18 \text{ patients}$$

To determine how many more patients would need to be on oxygen to reach the hospital policy amount, subtract the patients on oxygen now from the total.

$18 - 10 = 8$ more patients before oxygen would need to be requisitioned.

36. **The answer is a.** First convert the decimal amounts to whole numbers by multiplying them both by 100 and thus move the decimal point two places to the left.

$0.34 \overline{)86.36}$

will become

$34 \overline{)86.36} = 254.$

37. **The answer is b.** The larger negative addend allows you rewrite the problem with a negative sign, as it becomes a subtraction problem, despite the addition sign.

$22 - 19 =$ Solve the subtraction.

$22 - 19 = 3$ Determine if the answer should be negative or positive.

-3 The correct answer is -3.

The original addend (-22) was larger than the other addend $(+19)$.

38. **The answer is c.** You will have to borrow three times to answer this subtraction question.

39. **The answer is d.** Avoid concentrating on the hundredth digit and look instead to the thousandth digit. In this number, that would be 7, which is larger than 5, so you would round the hundredth digit 8 up to 9, and the thousandth and ten thousandth's digits would disappear. That would change 9,452.088 to 9,452.09.

40. **The answer is c.** You need to match the decimal place name to the denominator of the fraction on the right. Choice *a* has 3 in the tenths place, so it is false. Choice *b* has 48 in the thousandths place, so it is false. Choice *d* misstates the decimal place entirely. $11/6 = 1.83333333$. The correct answer has 294 in the ten thousandths place.

Science

1. **The answer is d.** Any combination that has the dominant (A) gene will display or show the trait, so the only combination that did not have the (A) gene and only an (a). Choice (d) is correct.

2. **The answer is c.** Each structural level is organized by function. The most basic is chemical, which is also the smallest. Molecules are made up by chemicals, and molecules form the cellular level. Cells form the tissue level, like muscle or nervous tissue. Tissues form the organ level. The stomach is one organ on this level and is part of the digestive system.

3. **The answer is d.** The humerus is one of the long bones of the leg. The sternum is a flat bone in the chest. The vertebra is an irregular bone in the back. The patella is a sesamoid bone in the knee.

4. **The answer is c.** Cl is more electronegative than H, so Cl pulls the shared pair of electrons to it, giving H a small positive charge; thus it is polar. The nonpolar covalent bonds are *a*, *b* (chlorine and hydrogen gas each sharing electrons equally), and *d* (methane gas).

5. **The answer is d.** Hyperventilation refers to excessive breathing that upsets the balance of carbon dioxide in the blood, causing lightheadedness. Hyperthermia is elevated body temperature. Hyperextension is movement beyond the normal range. Hypertonic describes a solution that causes cells to shrink through osmosis.

6. **The answer is c.** The scientists used two different sets of bacteria to show that while ordinary bacteria were mostly killed off by penicillin, those few that survived were not the cause of bacteria developing a resistance to penicillin over multiple generations. They used some bacteria whose forbearers had never been exposed to penicillin to show that bacteria could evolve with a resistance to bacteria due to other unknown factors.

7. **The answer is a.** The anther is part of the stamen, which is the male reproductive part of a flower. At its tip it holds the pollen in a sack just as the male testes in humans hold the sperm.

8. **The answer is d.** The ovary contains the ovule, which is a reproductive cell that becomes fertilized with pollen from the male flower. The stigma is the area of the female part of the flower that receives the pollen but does not produce seeds. The sepal is the base of the flower, and the peduncle is the stem. Neither of them is involved in reproduction.

9. **The answer is b.** The term for the speed achieved by a falling object as it is pulled to Earth by gravity is terminal velocity. The speed is limited by the drag or resistance applied to the object, which is the medium through which it is falling—in this case air. That speed can be 32 feet per second per second as it continuously falls. Gravitational attraction is only the description of a force on an object subject to mass attraction.

10. **The answer is b.** Five feet eight inches tall is 68 inches in height, and a weight of 153 is just over the 23 BMI ratio.

11. **The answer is c.** The BMI index shows that, at a BMI of 33 and a height of 76 inches, he would have to lose 66 pounds.

12. **The answer is d.** $KE = 1/2mv^2$. The velocity of an object is squared to calculate its kinetic energy. The energy of the car at 25 miles per hour was doubled, so its kinetic energy would quadruple.

13. **The answer is c.** The broadest form of classification is the domain. There are three domains that define all life: Bacteria, Archaea, and Eukarya, which include most of the living things commonly known and seen. The kingdoms are further divided into basics like animals, plants, fungi, and protists, which are all eukaryotic, and then archaea or bacteria, which are both microorganisms.

14. **The answer is d.** Parasites are organisms without a digestive system and rely upon a host to provide already digested food sources that they consume without permission. Tapeworms live in the intestines of organisms and feed off of already digested contents. Microorganisms in cows break down the sugar in cellulose, which cows can then digest. Remoras are in a symbiotic relationship with sharks that tolerate them because they clean the sharks and only eat bits of food sharks leave behind. Cows eating grass are consuming a primary food source and digesting it with microorganisms, not parasites.

15. **The answer is c.** In an emulsion, two liquids that are not soluble are mixed but do not break up or combine and remain suspended within each other. A tincture is a solution in which alcohol is the solvent.

16. **The answer is b.** The medulla oblongata regulates autonomic reflexes. The cerebrum controls voluntary movements. The cerebellum coordinates movements and cognition. The midbrain relays motor impulses.

17. **The answer is d.** The spinal cord sends nerve impulses to the skeletal muscles. The thalamus relays sensory input to the cerebral cortex. The cerebellum has other functions. The pons relays impulses between other parts of the brain.

18. **The answer is a.** The activated complex occurs at the moment of unstable arrangements of atoms, which results in the reformation of reactants and formation of products. The activation energy is B, which provides the energy for particles to react. The energy released by the reaction is C, which is the by-product of the reaction. The energy of the products is D, which is the end result of the reaction and the energy level of the products.

19. **The answer is b.** The rest of the graph would remain the same, but the curve of the activation energy would be far lower due to the fact that less energy would be needed with a catalyst. The activation complex would progress the same, and the same amount of energy would be released by the reaction and the products would have the same energy level at the end.

20. **The answer is c.** In this food web, snakes have only two food sources, rabbits and mice. If mice were much harder to find, snakes would only have rabbits to prey upon. Hawks would still have rabbits and snakes to prey upon. Rabbits and wildflowers don't prey on mice, so they would be unaffected.

21. **The answer is b.** The arrows indicate energy flow by having the base or start of a chain begin with an organism that is preyed upon and point to the organism that is consuming it.

22. **The answer is a.** Every organism would eventually be consumed by a decomposer after they die. Sunlight would only be consumed by producers like grass or wildflowers, which convert it to food. Sunlight itself is not consumed. Wolves are not primary consumers because they don't eat producers who create their own food from sunlight. Frogs could be secondary consumers of other organisms like insects that feed off of producers, but they do not eat grass.

23. **The answer is a.** The formula for sucrose or common table sugar describes 12 carbon atoms, 22 hydrogen atoms, and 11 oxygen atoms. Vinegar is b. Baking soda is c. Bleach is d.

24. **The answer is d.** A strong base like drain cleaner is at the extreme base end of the pH scale. 0 would be the exact opposite, like battery acid.

25. **The answer is c.** The chemical properties of an element change as you move from left to right in the table, not up and down. The entire table is arranged in increasing atomic number, not mass. The periods or rows correspond to principal energy levels.

26. **The answer is b.** The noble gases are stable, or inert, because their outermost electron shells are full.

27. **The answer is b.** The liver aids digestion by breaking down fats and detoxifying alcohol and drugs. The pancreas secretes pancreatic juices. The gallbladder stores bile and concentrates it. The colon completes digestion before expelling waste from the body.

28. **The answer is c.** The duodenum is the upper part of the small intestine. The appendix is a vestigial structure whose function is not certain. The ascending colon is the beginning of the large intestine, which processes food after the small intestine. The liver does not process or digest food directly.

29. **The answer is a.** Distal describes the position of one part relative to another such as a hand being farther away than attachment of a limb (an arm) to the trunk, at the shoulder. Proximal is closer to attachment to the trunk. Inferior describes away from the head or the lower part of the body, and posterior describes the back of the body.

30. **The answer is d.** "Water on the knee" is the name for delayed swelling that results from the body overproducing synovial fluid to help heal a knee injury resulting from torn menisci, or ligament sprains. The knee is not directly supported by muscles, only ligaments. After an injury, there may be some immediate swelling due to bleeding but not hours later. Dislocation would also cause swelling immediately.

31. **The answer is b.** Aluminum melts at 933 K and boils at 2,792 K. That's a difference of 1,850 K.

32. **The answer is d.** These Period 2 metals are not all metals. The first three are and thus melt and boil at lower temperatures.

33. **The answer is b.** Bases like soap have a slippery feel and taste bitter. Both acids and bases cause chemical dyes to change colors, but different colors. Only acids produce hydrogen when reacting with metals. Both acids and bases produce water and salt when reacting with hydroxide ions.

34. **The answer is d.** Boyle's law states that as the pressure of the gas increases and if the temperature is constant, the volume decreases. Charles's law is choice *a*. Gay-Lussac's law is choice *c*. And the combined gas law is choice *b*.

35. **The answer is c.** The vestibular apparatus is a series of channels, fluids, and hairs that provide equilibrium and balance. If overly stimulated by shock and sound waves, they will not function correctly and will create dizziness, or the body's inability to orient itself in space. The outer ear only collects sound to transmit it into the ear canal. The tympanic membrane vibrates when struck by sound waves,

which are interpreted by other nerves. The cochlea interprets sound waves into the sounds we hear.

36. **The answer is c.** Runners need carbohydrates for "carbo loading" as it's called. The purpose is to load up on energy in the form of glycogen, a highly branched molecule stored in the liver and muscles. Simple carbohydrates called monosaccharides are glucose and fructose found in such foods as pasta, bread, and rice. Lipids are fats and oils and are hard for the body to break down into energy. Cellulose is made up of plant sugars that few animals can digest. Amino acids are the building blocks of proteins, which provide some energy but not like carbohydrates can.

37. **The answer is b.** Trees cannot put down roots into the permafrost conditions of the tundra, where extremely cold temperatures keep the soil from fully thawing. Deserts are so dry that only a few types of trees can survive there, mostly around water sources. Conifers and other small trees can survive in the extreme cold of the taiga or boreal forests. Certain trees can live in the combination of grasslands and low rainfall called the savanna.

38. **The answer is d.** The electron microscope allows scientists to examine nanometer specimens. A pocket microscope is best used in the field for the examination of relatively large small objects. A compound microscope is best for laboratory examinations of slides. A digital microscope allows images to be recorded and sent from computer to computer.

39. **The answer is c.** The graph shows that after every hour, the car traveled 40 kilometers; so its speed is 40 km/hr.

40. **The answer is d.** The convenience comes from the decimal system, which deals in multiples of ten. People in the United States and a few other places are familiar with body temperature and freezing points in Fahrenheit readings, but the rest of the world is quite used to common Celsius temperature readings. The Fahrenheit scale has the advantage of more gradients over commonly used temperatures. Although a push was started in the United States in the 1970s to change over to the more universal metric system and Celsius, it never caught on, so Celsius must be converted to Fahrenheit and vice versa.

41. **The answer is c.** Amplitude is the height of a wave as shown in the distance described by C. The crest or high point of the wave is A. The low point or trough of the wave is B. The wavelength of a wave is the measurement of its movement until it returns to the same height or depth.

42. **The answer is d.** The frequency of a wave is counted by how often the crest of a wave passes a fixed point, in this case point A, in a second or any other measurement of time.

43. **The answer is c.** Humans cannot digest fiber in plants and fruits like apples and nuts, and this fiber helps get rid of bad cholesterol and keeps us regular. Fish is a good source of vitamins and minerals. Blueberries are an excellent source of phytochemicals, which promote health. Sweet potatoes are high in vitamin A, which helps your immune system.

44. **The answer is a.** The pyramid is older and still relies on more carbohydrates in the lowest level. The plate recommends equal amounts of grains and vegetables. The pyramid suggests about equal amounts of veggies and fruits, and so does the plate. The plate suggests different amounts of proteins and diary. The plate presents visual percentages for either a single meal or proportions for a whole diet. This is similar to the pyramid, which discusses multiple servings as a proportion.

45. **The answer is c.** Oils, fats, and sweets are not shown in the plate diagram because their percentage should be much smaller than the other major food groups. Dairy is shown as milk, yogurt, and cheese in the pyramid. Fruits are shown in both diagrams. Pasta is shown as grains in both, and nuts are listed as poultry in both.

46. **The answer is a.** A person whose heart has stopped is technically dead, so whatever risks would be involved in moving them have to be taken, with whatever precautions or stabilization possible. CPR only is necessary, not mouth-to-mouth.

47. **The answer is c.** Because this plant existed on the same level as an animal whose age has already been established, the age of the plant can also be established. The fact that the plant existed deeper doesn't change the dating of the animal's age. The date of extinction of the plant cannot be determined unless multiple samples showed that it wasn't found at the age of those digs. The fact that the plant is older doesn't change the known date of the animal.

48. **The answer is d.** Budding, miotic cell division, and clones are all asexual reproduction. Gametes, male and female cells, are only produced during sexual reproduction.

49. **The answer is a.** A tree grows in width through the action of cambium cells known as xylem and phloem. The inner layer of the bark continues to grow even when the center is dead. The xylem is woody tissue that supports the trunk and brings water to the whole tree. The phloem supplies food to the tree. As long as these cells continue to function, a hollow tree can live.

50. **The answer is b.** As a cycle, water that comes out of the atmosphere and falls to Earth as precipitation has to have some means by which it could be returned to the atmosphere. Without evaporation, water would not rise from the ground or water sources to create clouds or saturate the atmosphere. Groundwater is precipitation or underground water that does not depend on evaporation. Rain and snow soak into the ground due to gravity, not evaporation. Respiration in plants is gas being released into the atmosphere. For the cycle to be truly circular, all parts are necessary.

51. **The answer is d.** Without a control step, the student would not have any proven base amount of acid in the air in the bag before exercising to compare with the amount of acid in the air in the bag after exercise. The hypothesis is clearly stated in proving that CO_2 content in exhaled air increases during exercise. Measuring the acid content in the exhaled air by bubbling it through water is a testing step. The repeat step would be done by other students or scientists verifying any results of this experiment.

52. **The answer is d.** The first action to be taken on a triage scene is to treat injuries or wounds that could result in death without easily applied measures and techniques. Heavy loss of blood can kill quickly, and direct pressure or a tourniquet can stop blood flow relatively easily and save lives. Burns that are second degree to 30 percent of the body or third degree to 10 percent are serious but fall into the second tier of triage unless the air passages are damaged, which would be first priority. Identifying those who need hospitalization or those who are so badly injured as to be near death or dead are secondary issues to address.

53. **The answer is c.** All these statements are true except the fact that permanent effects of drug addiction can be avoided. It is a brain disorder that affects reward, self-control, and stress even after an addiction has been controlled.

54. **The answer is d.** Animal or plant cells are small parts of a larger multicellular organism. An amoeba is a single cell that is a complete organism not acting together with other similar cells to form a larger organism. It does have cytoplasm and a vacuole.

55. **The answer is b.** The organisms in Chordata, such as mammals, birds, reptiles, amphibians, and fish, have some form of a spinal cord and nervous system. Many different phyla have bilateral symmetry and a separate mouth and anus. Annelida or worms have ringed specialized segments.

56. **The answer is a.** The lymphatic system is part of the body's natural defenses against outside contamination by circulating lymph to provide immunity. The respiratory system (b) deals with gas and heat exchange through breathing. The digestive system (c) takes in food, which it converts into needed chemicals. The circulatory system (d) moves blood throughout the body, pumped by the heart.

57. **The answer is b.** Skeletal muscle tissues have the longest type of fibers in order to contract and expand over longer ranges to move long bones. Cardiac tissue fibers are short and dense (50 to 100 microns) for intense and repetitive contractions, while the smooth muscle of internal organs and blood vessels are more in the median range (20 to 500 microns) for a variety of functions. No muscle tissue is 100 to 200 cm long.

58. **The answer is d.** The mitochondria (d) produce ATP as an energy source. Muscle cells have many mitochondria. The cytoplasm of intracellular fluid is contained by

the (b) plasma membrane that surrounds the cell. The nucleus (c) contains DNA and other genetic material. The Golgi complex (a) makes proteins of various sorts available to the cell.

59. **The answer is a.** In cellular respiration of animals, oxygen (O_2) is taken in and carbon dioxide (CO_2) and water (H_2O) are released as waste products.

60. **The answer is a.** Osmosis describes water molecules passing through a semipermeable barrier such as a cell wall through openings too small for other molecules to pass through. They move into areas of higher concentration to dilute it. Diffusion describes water molecules moving within a solution to balance concentrations. Active transport describes a chemical transfer using energy to move molecules through a cell wall. Transpiration describes the release of water vapor from plants into the atmosphere.

Note

Note

Note

Note

Note

Note

Note

Note

Note

Note

Note